THE NURSE
AS MANAGER

THE NURSE
AS MANAGER⟩

Joyce L. Schweiger, R.N., M.S.
University of Delaware, Newark

A WILEY MEDICAL PUBLICATION
JOHN WILEY & SONS
New York • Chichester • Brisbane • Toronto

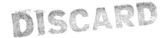

Cover design: Wanda Lubelska
Production editor: Cheryl Howell

Library of Congress Cataloging in Publication Data

Main entry under title:
The nurse as manager

  Includes index
  1. Nursing service administration. 2. Communica-
tion in nursing. I. Schweiger, Joyce L.
[DNLM: 1. Communication. 2. Nursing, Supervisory.
WY105 S413m]
RT89.M36   610.73′068   80-17456
ISBN 0-471-04343-5

Printed in the United States of America

10 9 8 7 6 5 4 3 2 1

Contributors

Dorothy A. Kennedy, R.N., M.A.
Associate Professor Maternal/Child Nursing
University of Delaware College of Nursing
Newark, Delaware

Mary Lou Hamilton, R.N., M.S.
Assistant Professor Psychiatric/Mental Health Nursing
University of Delaware College of Nursing
Newark, Delaware

Mary Ann Miller, R.N., M.S.N.
Assistant Professor Maternal/Child Nursing
University of Delaware College of Nursing
Newark, Delaware

Malinda Murray, R.N., M.Ed.
Chairperson and Associate Professor
West Chester State College, Department of Nursing
West Chester, Pennsylvania

Anthony J. Spinato, F.H.F.M.A.
Controller
Community General Hospital
Reading, Pennsylvania

Preface

Just as the nurse's role has expanded in relation to patient care responsibilities, so has it expanded in relation to management functions. But little attention has been paid to the nurse's role as manager compared with that paid to the expanded role of the nurse practitioner or clinical specialist. Therefore, nurses, who comprise the single largest group of health care providers, often find themselves placed in management positions for which they have had little formal or informal preparation.

The purpose of this book is to help resolve this problem by providing practicing nurses and professional nursing students with a practical guide to management knowledge, skills, and techniques as they apply to practice in clinical agencies. My intention is to help ease the transition from the role of nursing student to nurse-manager or from staff nurse to nursing supervisor, head nurse, or nursing administrator, by preparing the reader for some of the realities of practice. I also hope to increase the reader's awareness of the many factors that determine how effectively he or she will function in a management role. Throughout the book, actual situations from various practice settings—situations with which the reader can readily identify—are included to illustrate points made in the text.

Chapters 1 through 4 provide an introduction to basic management theory and the subject of accountability. The principles in these chapters constitute a foundation for the specific topics addressed later in the book. Chapter 1 gives an overview of the major philosophies, objectives, and policies of health care agencies, knowledge the nurse-manager must have about the institution where he or she works in order to help carry out its goals. In Chapter 2 the basic organizational structures of health care agencies are explained. Understanding the chain of command is essential to effective functioning as a manager. Quality assurance and accountability, the subjects of Chapter 3, are receiving increasing attention because of consumer demands for better health care, rising health care costs, and federal intervention. Chapter 4 describes not only the various basic styles of leadership but also the variables that control these styles. Chapter 5 explores communication skills — oral, written, and nonverbal — and the importance of these skills in functioning successfully as a manager.

Chapters 6 through 9 cover topics that personally involve both the nurse-manager and the nursing staff and that have a direct bearing on the quality of patient care. In Chapter 6 the seven basic steps in problem solving are discussed. The importance of thoroughly investigating the facts before trying to resolve a problem is emphasized. Chapter 7 describes the influences that stimulate or hinder change and how strengths are maximized and forces of resistance are minimized in situations of planned change. Chapter 8 on staff motivation catalogues thirteen ways the nurse-manager can motivate staff members to accept increasing responsibility for improving patient care. Chapter 9 addresses the topics of staffing patterns and factors that affect staffing decisions.

The last four chapters of the book describe specific tools used by the nurse in order to function effectively as a manager in a health care agency. An entire chapter, Chapter 10, is devoted to job descriptions because practicing nurses often ignore this essential determinant of their accountability and scope of practice. How to write a good job description is included. Staff evaluation, an important managerial function, is the subject of Chapter 11. Staff evaluation for job promotion, change, and termination is carefully distinguished from patient care evaluation in quality assurance programs. Chapter 12 offers detailed descriptions of how to prepare a nursing budget. The final chapter of the book examines labor-management relations, an increasingly important topic in view of the growing assertiveness and power of nurses in the health care system.

For the sake of simplicity and clarity, throughout the text I have used the feminine pronouns to refer to the nurse. No discrimination against male nurses is intended.

I wrote this book with the firm conviction that greater opportunities for expansion within management and leadership roles should be and will become available to professional nurses. These opportunities will help nurses establish their identity as professionals and will surely contribute to their greater vitality, productivity, and involvement in our health care system in the years to come.

Joyce L. Schweiger

Acknowledgments

There are many people to whom I would like to express my thanks and appreciation for the encouragement and support they provided me. I wish to begin by thanking my students, the practicing nurses, and workshop participants, who made me acutely aware of the need to provide a how-to approach to management problems. Their willingness to share their problems and frustrations provided the necessary catalyst to pursue the writing of this book.

I wish to especially thank Mary Ann Miller, a colleague in nursing education, for her continued support and inspiring suggestions related to the major content of the book. My appreciation is extended to Corrine Price and Marjorie Recke for their endeavors in researching material and sharing ideas that were incorporated in the chapters on communication, leadership, and change. Thanks to Donald E. Glasford, Administrator, Community General Hospital, Reading, Pennsylvania, for his suggestions and critique of Chapter 13 on labor relations.

I am especially grateful to Russel C. Swansburg, Associate Professor and Acting Chairman, Medical Surgical Nursing, at the University of South Alabama, for giving me permission to use an extensive amount of his material related to Chapter 10, Job Descriptions. Also thanks to Ruth Kirkman, Director of Nursing, Crozier-Chester Medical Center, Chester, Pennsylvania, for allowing me to use the basic concepts of the nurse supervisor's job description as a framework to illustrate the job description format.

The illustrations in Chapters 5, 10, and 12 that have clarified and emphasized issues were contributed by Jan Spinato, Allentown, Pennsylvania.

Preparation of this book would not have been possible without the typing and refinement of details that were provided by Anne Downey, Ramona Denn, Barbara McKinney, and Diane Miller.

Finally, the greatest thanks and appreciation to my husband Jim, who encouraged me and put up with all my mood swings, particularly during the concluding months and weeks of the manuscript's preparation.

Joyce L. Schweiger

Contents

1. **Philosophy, Objectives, Policies, and Procedures
    of Health Care Agencies**
    "The Beginning"
    Dorothy A. Kennedy   1

2. **Organizational Structure of Health Care Agencies**   13
    "Pyramids and Parallelograms"
    Malinda Murray

3. **Quality Assurance and Accountability in Health
    Care Delivery**
    "Cope With or Cop Out"   23
    Joyce L. Schweiger

4. **Leadership Styles**   37
    "Be a Leader, Not a Boss"
    Joyce L. Schweiger and Mary Lou Hamilton

5. **Inter- and Intradepartmental Communication**   50
    "Tune In or Tune Out"
    Joyce L. Schweiger

6. **Problem Solving**   63
    "An Active Exercise"
    Joyce L. Schweiger

7. **Change Without Disruption**   75
    "The Need to Plan Ahead"
    Mary Ann Miller

8. **Staff Motivation**   **87**
   "A Rolling Stone . . . ?"
   Mary Lou Hamilton

9. **Staffing and Staffing Patterns**   **104**
   "A Jigsaw Puzzle"
   Joyce L. Schweiger

10. **Job Descriptions**   **118**
    "Vital Statistics"
    Joyce L. Schweiger

11. **Staff Evaluation**   **131**
    "Pain or Pleasure"
    Mary Ann Miller

12. **Fiscal Planning**   **144**
    "To Have or Have Not"
    Anthony J. Spinato

13. **Labor-Management Relations in Health Care Delivery**   **168**
    "A Basic Understanding"
    Joyce L. Schweiger

   Appendix A. Job Descriptions (Sample)   **181**

   Appendix B. Patient Questionnaire (Sample)   **187**

   Index   **191**

THE NURSE
AS MANAGER

1. Philosophy, Objectives, Policies, and Procedures of Health Care Agencies

"The Beginning"

Dorothy A. Kennedy, R.N., M.A.

BEHAVIORAL OBJECTIVES

After reviewing this chapter, the reader will be able to

- identify the relationship between the purpose of goals of health care agencies and the philosophy, objectives, policies, and procedures of the agency
- describe the components of the philosophy of a nursing department
- identify the differences between structure, process, and outcome objectives
- compare and contrast objectives classified on a temporal continuum with objectives classified as maintenance change
- describe the relationship of policies and procedures to objectives
- identify the key characteristics of useful policies

A nurse who accepts a position in a health care agency makes a commitment to the goals and philosophy of the organization and to the philosophy of nursing care within the organization. A nurse who accepts an appointment to a management position in the department of nursing not only makes the same commitment but also must subscribe to the philosophy of management endorsed by the department. The pledge may be tacit or overt; nevertheless, it is made. It is essential, therefore, that nurses become aware of the goals and philosophy of the agency with which they are associated or in which they are seeking a position.

Peterson (1) draws a conceptual distinction between the words *purpose* and *goal*. He refers to *purpose* as the stated mission of types of institutions. Applying his definition of *purpose* to health care institutions, one would speak of the purpose of types of agencies such as visiting nurse association, Veterans Administration hospitals, community hospitals, and crisis centers. In Peterson's conceptual framework, *goal* refers to specified ends of a particular institution. Although all community hospitals may have the same purpose, each community hospital has its own set of goals.

Cantor (2), in her succinct discussion of philosophy, purpose, and objectives for nursing departments, uses the word *purpose* to refer to the specified reason for the existence of a particular health care agency and of each department, including nursing, within that agency. Throughout this chapter, the words *goal* and *purpose* are used interchangeably.

PURPOSE

The purpose of a health care agency may have been set forth when the institution was established and may have remained relatively unchanged over the years. On the other hand, a health care agency must be responsive to external as well as internal forces if it is to continue to exist; therefore, goals may be modified in time. Visiting nurse associations have shifted from exclusively home-based nursing services to home based health care services and have added other health professionals to a staff previously composed only of nurses. A hospital chartered to provide general medical and surgical care in an urban-suburban area may evolve into a tertiary care center serving a much larger geographic region. A health care agency established primarily to provide direct services to clients may eventually become primarily a teaching center for health professionals. It is the responsibility of the board of trustees or directors of a health care agency to set the goals for the agency with input and advice from agency administrators, including the chief nursing administrator, and from the consumers of its services.

The broad purposes or goals of a health care agency are usually available as a printed document, because most agencies depend on external sources for some or all of their operating funds. Fund-raising

brochures or annual reports are prepared to inform people outside the
agency about the goals of the agency and the contributions it makes to
the health and well being of the citizens in the area it serves. The
purpose of a nursing department within a health care agency is derived from the broad goals of the agency and must be consistent with
those goals.

Too frequently, nurses and others in an agency assume that the only
purpose of the nursing department is to deliver nursing care of the
highest quality to the clients of the agency, even though the agency
declares in its goal statement that education of health professionals,
research related to health and illness, and health education for the
citizens it serves are also among the major purposes of the institution.
The nursing department should have a clear statement of purpose that
specifies the department's contribution to the purposes of the institution of which it is a part. Each subunit within the nursing department
should also have a statement of purpose that delineates the part the
particular unit is expected to play in achieving the goals of that department and, by doing so, the purposes of the health care agency as a
whole.

PHILOSOPHY

An organizational philosophy is a set of beliefs that determines how
organizational purposes are achieved and that serves as the foundation for agency objectives, policies, and procedures. Although the artic-
ulation of beliefs in the form of a statement of philosophy has long
been advocated for educational programs in general and for nursing
education programs in particular, less significance has been attached
to the delineation of beliefs underlying the administration of health
care agencies. Many nurses have been required to write a statement of
their philosophy of nursing at some point during their educational
program and have been impressed with the need to make explicit beliefs that underlie action. These same nurses are dismayed when they
find that a health care agency does not have a written statement of
philosophy that serves as the framework for the philosophy of its nursing department. The lack of an institutional statement of philosophy
should not deter the nursing department from formulating such a
statement. Nurses have a right to know the beliefs about nursing care,
nursing practice, and nursing management held by the collective
group of which they are a part—the nursing department. A statement

of philosophy that is not just a collection of words and phrases currently or perennially bandied about but is grounded in actions is a valuable management tool. Nurses should be given a copy before they join the staff so that they can judge whether their personal philosophy is sufficiently in agreement with the organizational philosophy to enable them to become a contributing member of the department.

DiVincenti (3, p. 85) lists 17 concepts culled from a review of the philosophy statements of 80 nursing departments. She defends the idealistic quality of nursing department statements of philosophy on the grounds that aiming at superior performance and perfection stimulates outstanding progress. Cantor (2, p. 11) emphasizes that the philosophy of the nursing department should address only those concerns directly relevant to the collective group of individuals who comprise the nursing department. It is the patient who receives the service of the health care agency; thus it is the nursing care required by the patient that should be addressed in the philosophy of the department. Additional beliefs that should be treated in the philosophy statement are the beliefs about nursing management. A review of philosophy statements of nursing departments (3, pp.335–342) reveals that beliefs related to management are reflected, if at all, in global terms such as "promote a working environment conducive to the growth of all persons," or "employees are persons of dignity and worth and must be given the opportunity to develop." The philosophy of nursing service included by Martel (4) in an article in *Nursing Administration Quarterly* contains a statement related more specifically to nursing management. The statement indicates that decision making by the practitioner is sufficiently important that the organizational structure and style of leadership must facilitate the decision process in direct nurse-client encounters.

The collective group that is the department of nursing within a health care agency may consist only of nurses with the same level of educational preparation—for example, a community service for families of children with developmental disabilities staffed by nurse specialists with master's degrees in nursing, or a city, county, or state public health nursing service that employs only nurses with baccalaureate degrees in nursing. On the other hand, the group may consist of people with widely divergent experience and educational preparation—for example, people whose formal education in nursing ranges from on-the-job training to doctoral study in nursing science or in a discipline related to nursing. A philosophy of nursing management should include beliefs about levels of practice, responsibility, and accountability expected of the several levels of practitioners in the group. Such beliefs are held by members of the nursing department and should be expressed so that the philosophy can be useful in guiding all members in the achievement of departmental goals.

If the philosophy of the nursing department is to serve as a common point of reference for all members, it must be phrased in words that clearly express the beliefs of the group. It is more useful if the philosophy is developed as a list of individual statements of belief grouped under the separate headings of nursing care, nursing practice, and nursing management. In this form, beliefs will stand out as separate entities and will not be buried as they might be in a document written in narrative style. The statement must deal with specifics related to the purposes of the department, not with generalizations. Also it must be sufficiently inclusive to serve as a framework from which the philosophy statement of each unit within the nursing department can be drawn.

Although each unit within the nursing department supports the philosophy of the department, it must also set forth its beliefs regarding nursing care, nursing practice, and nursing management on the unit. The types of patients, the levels of nursing personnel, and functions differ among units; therefore, the set of beliefs that underlies the actions of the collective group on each unit should be developed. The philosophy of a pediatric unit that provides rooming-in facilities for parents would differ somewhat from that of a medical unit for adult clients. The philosophy of a home care unit would differ from that of an inpatient unit.

Philosophy statements are relatively enduring documents because stated beliefs are usually expressions of firm commitment to the best that can be achieved and are derived from the broad goals of the agency. Norris (5) points out that a useful philosophy has a timeless quality because basic premises change only under unusual conditions. Nevertheless, philosophy statements need to be reviewed periodically. Just as a work tool needs inspection, and perhaps sharpening, from time to time, so does a management tool. If a review by all members of the department reveals that the statement still reflects the guiding beliefs of the collective group, there is no need to revise the document. If close scrutiny indicates that the statement is not consistent with current agency goals or philosophy or is not effective in directing the actions of the department, then the statement should be rewritten to assure that it meets the criteria of compatibility, attainability, intelligibility, acceptability, measureability, and accountability (6).

OBJECTIVES

Abstract concepts are the building blocks of statements of goals and philosophy. Objectives are statements of concrete results to be achieved in order that the goals can be reached. Just as the goals and philosophy of the nursing department are drawn from the more global goals and philosophy of the health care agency, so too are the nursing department objectives related to the objectives of the organization (see Fig. 1-1). Objectives for all levels of the health care agency can be classified in several ways. Objectives can be categorized as "structure," "process," or "outcome" statements.

Structure objectives relate to the framework in which an activity is carried out, e.g., "The nursing department provides a continuous edu-

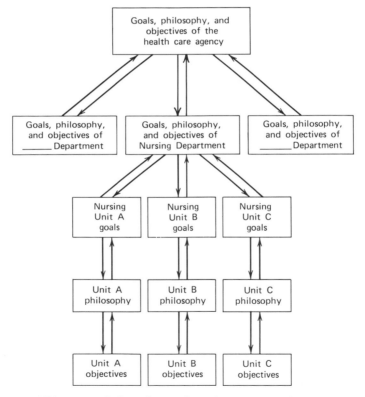

Figure 1-1. Diagram of the relationship of institutional goals, philosophy, and objectives to those of departments and of units within the nursing department.

cational program to assure competency of all registered nurses in administering medication."

Process statements specify the methods to be used to achieve results, e.g., "Registered nurses attend a refresher program in administration of medications every twelve months." A review of published statements of nursing departments (3, pp. 335–342; 4, p. 13) indicates that the objectives can be classified most frequently as process objectives.

Outcome objectives, on the other hand, delineate the ends to be attained through the activities of the organization and its many subunits. An outcome objective for a nursing department might be "Patients learn the purpose, ordered amount, time schedule, and period of administration of medications ordered by their physicians." Cantor (2, p. 12) stresses that focusing on methods rather than on results can lead to continuation of nursing interventions that are ineffective in achieving desired ends.

DiVincenti (3, pp. 93–94) proposes a classification of objectives along a temporal continuum: permanent, long-range, and short-range. Permanent objectives or ideals are statements of the optimal results that an organization, or one or more of its subunits, strives to achieve — enduring, basic, hoped-for outcomes of the activities of the organization. Long-range objectives set forth the results to be achieved over an extended period, often three to five years — statements that are derived from the permanent objectives. Short-range objectives are specific outcomes of activity within a limited time span, usually 6 to 12 months, and are programmed steps toward the attainment of long-range objectives.

Permanent, long-range, and short-range objectives expressed as outcomes play a major role in a philosophy and method of management proposed by Drucker (7) as "management by objectives" (MBO). This method is a process designed to involve managers at all levels of an organization in setting objectives, planning action to achieve the objectives, determining who is responsible for producing the results, measuring the attainment of the results at specified points in time, and assessing each person's contribution to the results (8,9). The MBO approach is results-oriented and is based on the concept that employees who know in detail the objectives of the organization and their expected contribution toward attaining the results not only will be more productive but also will achieve more personal satisfaction in their position.

Statements of objectives, regardless of type, should be clear and concise and should be written in terms related specifically to the outcomes to be achieved. In health care agencies, the results expected on nursing units are changes in the clients or patients and in those persons who provide the care. The objectives should be realistic and yet stimulate movement toward higher standards of care and employee growth. Objectives should be measurable and, whenever possible, quantifiable. Objectives for the individual nursing units can be more specific than objectives for the entire nursing department. Because of the complexity of the goals of most nursing departments, some of the objectives of the department and its units cannot be met without assistance from and cooperation with departments within the agency. It is essential, therefore, that the contribution of each department be specified and that there be mutual objective setting and planning.

Sherwin (10) proposes the use of an objectives grid to identify the positions and the persons whose contributions are required to achieve each objective. Although his example applies to objectives set for an agency as a whole, the concept is applicable at the department and unit level. Sherwin also presents another classification of objectives — performance maintenance objectives and change or improvement objectives. To achieve maintenance objectives, employees follow well-established guidelines and procedures proven effective in attaining desired results. Change objectives require new or modified behaviors on the part of employees. In addition, policy changes, new equipment, or personnel changes may be required to meet change objectives. Viewing objectives from a maintenance-change perspective enables those who set objectives to be realistic and yet creative in the objectives set for the unit and to focus on the existing strengths of the unit.

POLICIES AND PROCEDURES

Objectives set forth the ends toward which an organization is striving; policies and procedures are guidelines to be followed in the pursuit of the ends. Policies are guidelines for decisions about actions; procedures are directions for actions. In an organization there are policies and procedures that apply to every department or unit within the organization, and there are some that are specific to the objectives of the individual unit. In health care agencies, policies related to the protection of the rights of clients and their families and to the safety of personnel are examples of overall agency policies; policies on the administration of medications are nursing department policies, whereas policies on the prescription of medications are medical department policies. A policy on informed consent for treatment would be the same for every department involved in providing care, but the procedure to be followed in the emergency room might be different, at least in part, from the procedure for inpatient units.

Although policies may seem to be designed to constrain action, they free individuals to act without having to examine the benefits and risks inherent in each of the alternatives for action. Many people view policies negatively because of past experience with outdated, excessively restrictive, or inoperable policies. Others recognize that policies make a positive contribution to the achievement of objectives because, without useful policies, inconsistencies and inequalities would abound.

What are the characteristics of a useful policy? Moore (11) states that a clear statement of purpose for each policy is essential. Is the policy designed to protect client welfare, to safeguard the rights of the client and his family, to protect or satisfy employee needs, or to maximize the utilization of fiscal, material, or personnel resources? Unless the purpose of the policy is delineated, one cannot judge the degree to which the policy contributes to the attainment of the objectives of the organization.

Another key characteristic of a useful policy is a clear or specific statement of who can implement the policy. A nursing department policy on the administration of medications on general medical and surgical units might specify that registered nurses and licensed practical nurses can administer oral medications ordered on a scheduled dosage—for example, four times a day or every eight hours, but that oral p.r.n. medications are to be administered only by the nurse-in-charge.

Applicability of the policy in the setting for which it is intended is another key characteristic of a useful policy. An overall personnel policy for a health care agency that states that every employee is entitled to have two consecutive days off each week may be applicable in some departments all the time, in some departments part of the time, and in other departments rarely, if ever. The fact that the policy is not upheld in some departments indicates either that the policy should be changed or that changes need to be made in the scheduling procedure or in the personnel of the departments in which the policy is not implemented. A pediatric unit might have a policy that states that two nurses are to be present when an intramuscular injection is given to any child under eight years of age. One nurse is to hold and support the child while the other nurse administers the medication. In practice, the policy is applicable on the day and evening tours because there are always at least two nurses on the unit. On the night tour, however, there is only one nurse. To adhere to the policy, the nurse must call a nurse from another unit or the nursing supervisor. On the other hand, the nurse may decide to adhere only to the intent of the policy, and not to specific features, by asking a parent or relative to hold the child.

In assessing the applicability of the policy, its purpose must be reviewed. If the purpose is to provide a qualified witness in the event of an injury to the child from the injection, then the policy as worded should remain and the staffing of the night tours should be changed. If the purpose is to protect the physical and emotional welfare of the child, and if the nurses are judged to have the ability to assess the situation and make provision for the welfare of the child, then the policy could be changed to allow the nurse to decide whether or not assistance is needed and, if so, from whom.

A policy is useful only if it is known to those who are expected to adhere to it. It must be written in terms intelligible to the people it is intended to guide; it must be communicated to them; and it must be available for reference when needed. Policies that guide the actions of members of the nursing department should be available, in up-to-date form, in manuals on each nursing unit. Each manual should have a table of contents and an index. Every policy statement should include the date of its establishment and the authorizing group within the organization or department. Any statement established because of stipulations of an external authority – for example, licensing board, funding agency, or court decision – should include documentation of that source also.

In health care agencies where one or more departments provide service 24 hours a day, 7 days a week, communication about policy additions, revisions, or deletions is more difficult than in agencies where all or most personnel maintain the same work schedule. Notices posted on bulletin boards, announcements at change-of-tour reports, and notices circulated from person to person within a unit or department have been used with some degree of success to keep employees abreast of policy changes. Greater success has been gained from the inclusion in each person's pay envelope of notice of changes.

Perhaps more difficult than the development of a useful policy is the maintenance of a functional policy manual. Unless some person or group within an organization and its departments is charged with auditing the policy statements and their effectiveness in guiding people in the achievement of expected outcomes, a manual can become a repository of outmoded or inadequate documents. Not only does a policy manual have to be viewed as a guide for employees, it must also be recognized as a protection for the health care agency and as evidence of quality of care. Policy manuals may be referred to in instances in which there are differences of opinion between health care providers and consumers. Policy manuals are also references used by external authorities in the process of licensure or certification review. It is essential, then, that maintenance of functional manuals be one of the top priorities of nurse-managers.

Procedures elaborate the steps to be taken to implement a policy or to complete a task. A useful procedure has the same characteristics as a useful policy — purpose, specificity of actor, applicability to the setting, as well as intelligibility or communicability. Procedures must be monitored with the same vigor as policies. Because procedure descriptions are tools used not only to refresh the memory of continuing employees but also to teach new employees, they must contain enough detail to be useful in orientation and training. Because procedures are used as teaching tools, care should be taken to document, whenever possible, the references used in preparing a procedure description.

Although the nurse-manager relies heavily upon policies and procedures in day-to-day actions, the goals, philosophy, and objectives of the health care agency and of the nursing department influence actions. Objectives reflect goals and philosophy; policy and procedures are the guidelines used by nurse-managers to meet their responsibility to attain expected outcomes.

REFERENCES

1. Peterson RE: *The Crisis of Purpose: Definition and Uses of Institutional Goals.* Princeton, NJ, Educational Testing Service, 1970, p. 3.
2. Cantor MM: Philosophy, purpose, and objectives: why do we have them? *J Nurs Adm* 1:9–14, May-June 1971.
3. DiVincenti M: *Administering Nursing Service,* ed 2. Boston, Little Brown & Co, 1977, p. 85.
4. Martel GD: On the scene: organizational structures of nursing services at Northwestern Memorial Hospital: the organizational system. *Nurs Adm Q* 3:12, Winter 1979.
5. Norris CM: Building a useful philosophy of nursing, in Zderad LT, Belcher, H (eds): *Developing Behavioral Concepts in Nursing.* Atlanta, Southern Regional Education Board, 1968, p. 104.
6. Bolin JG: Six criteria for better goals, in *Improving College and University Teaching* 21:245, 1973.
7. Drucker P: *People and Performance: The Best of Peter Drucker on Management.* New York, Harper & Row, 1977, pp. 64–66, 119–121.

8. Palmer J: Management by objectives. *J Nurs Adm* 1:17–23, January 1971.
9. Cain C, Luchsinger V: Management by objectives: applications to nursing. *J Nurs Adm* 8:35–38, January 1978.
10. Sherwin DS: Management of objectives. *Harvard Bus Rev* 54:151, May-June 1976.
11. Moore M: Standard 3: policies . . . guidelines for action. *J Nurs Adm* 2:31, May-June 1972.

BIBLIOGRAPHY

Periodicals

Boissoneau R: The nursing human service administrator. *Nurs Adm Q* 3:1–9, Winter 1979.
Marriner A: Development of management thought. *J Nurs Adm* 9:21–31, September, 1979.
McClure ML: The administrative component of the nurse administrator's role. *Nurs Adm Q* 3:1–12, Summer 1979.

Books

Beyers M, Phillips C: *Nursing Management for Patient Care,* ed 2. Boston, Little Brown & Co, 1979.
Clark CG, Shea CA: *Management in Nursing: A Vital Link in the Health Care System.* New York, McGraw-Hill Book Co, 1979.
Ganong JM, Ganong WL: *Nursing Management: Concepts, Functions, Techniques, and Skills.* Germantown, Md, Aspen Systems Corp, 1976.
Raia AP: *Managing by Objectives.* Glenview, Ill, Scott Foresman & Co, 1974.
Shanks MD, Kennedy DA: *Administracion y enfermeria,* ed 2. Mexico City, Nueva Editorial Interamericana, 1973.
Stevens BJ: *First-Line Patient Care Management.* Wakefield, Mass, Contemporary Publishing Inc, 1976.
Stevens WF: *Management and Leadership in Nursing.* New York, McGraw-Hill Book Co, 1978.
Stone S, et al (eds): *Management for Nurses: A Multidisciplinary Approach.* St Louis, The CV Mosby Co, 1976.

2. Organizational Structure of Health Care Agencies

"Pyramids and Parallelograms"

Malinda Murray, R.N., M.Ed.

BEHAVIORAL OBJECTIVES

After reviewing this chapter, the reader will be able to

- identify and describe a variety of organizational structures, both formal and informal
- describe the lines of authority and influence within health care agencies
- compare and contrast line and staff positions
- use the knowledge of organizational structure to improve individual effectiveness and the quality of patient care

Many staff nurses view the organizational structure of health care agencies as a maze within which they energetically search for the path to their goal of providing quality patient care; instead, they find themselves continually running into dead ends. Under these circumstances, good ideas are often lost because ineffective routes are used in passing these ideas along to the appropriate person or because the wrong person is selected as the recipient of the ideas. Frequently, the staff nurses then become frustrated and begin to believe that administrators are not interested in their contributions. These nurses are likely to criticize the agency structure itself because, they insist, it "stifles creativity" and "cramps style."

In this situation, the agency structure is seen as a series of barriers that have to be overcome before anything useful can be accomplished. However, when observed from a bird's-eye view, a maze can suddenly become a map, a useful tool that facilitates progress toward a goal.

REASONS FOR STRUCTURE

There are three main reasons for having an organizational structure, based on the fundamental need to bring order to the official relationships among all employees so that they can work effectively and systematically together. The first reason is to delineate levels of authority. It is essential for all employees to know to whom they are responsible and for whom they are responsible, especially as the number of people within a level increases. Much of the frustration that nurses experience is due to the fact that too many different people are giving them directions, that expectations of their work are inadequately explained, or that their authority and accountability regarding the work of other personnel are not well defined. When levels of authority are clearly delineated and functioning well, the chances for personal satisfaction and effectiveness for everyone concerned, including the patient, are markedly increased.

The second reason for an organization to have a designated structure is to reduce duplication of effort. A division of labor identifies subgroups in relation to special interests or skills. Within the subgroups, levels of authority are described. The reason for division of labor is to use material and personnel resources most efficiently by having those most skilled in a specific area carrying out essential tasks. One approach to division of labor is departmentalization within the hospital, where each department is expected to deliver a particular specialized function such as pharmacological services, physical therapy, outpatient care, or storage and retrieval of patient records.

The third reason for organizational structure is to identify channels of communication, horizontally as well as vertically. In the traditional structure, most communication was from the top down, in the form of rules, policies, and directives issued by superiors to subordinates. However, with the current trend toward greater participation in decision making by staff at all levels, communications are now rising from bottom to top as well. Better communication within the same level is also recognized as very useful.

LINE AND STAFF RELATIONSHIPS

Within an organization, certain basic types of relationships must be understood in the context of the institutional structure. These relationships may cut across levels of authority, divisions of labor, and channels of communication. The kinds of relationships most frequently encountered are called *line* and *staff*. (Note that in this context *staff* has a much different meaning than in the phrase *staff nurse*.)

People in line positions are those who are links in the chain of command, who are directly responsible and accountable for accomplishing the objectives of the agency. These people make decisions that affect the agency and its goals. They enforce agency policies and guide and evaluate their subordinates. Staff personnel, in contrast, are the support groups that make it possible for the agency to reach its goals. They function in an advisory capacity only, offering suggestions to those who actually make the decisions that affect the agency. The power of staff personnel lies in "friendly persuasion" and in the respect they command (usually because of expertise), since they are not in a direct line of delegated authority.

In a health care agency, the use of both line and staff positions in nursing is a long-established tradition, with the nursing director, associate and assistant directors, supervisors, and head nurses in line positions of successive levels of authority, ultimately over the group of nurses and auxiliary nursing personnel providing direct daily patient care. The concept of staff positions in nursing, however, is sometimes less easily identified. The idea of the staff role for nurses is much newer and has developed with the growing demands of nurses for professional autonomy. With the variety of expanded nursing roles in all kinds of health care settings, the controversy over how to define the positions of clinical nurse specialists and nurse practitioners has yet to be resolved completely. At the present time, each agency determines for itself whether these specialists will assume a line or staff role, or a combination of both.

FORMAL ORGANIZATIONAL STRUCTURES: PYRAMID AND MATRIX

Work-oriented institutions may be set up according to any of several types of formal organizational structures, as well as by developing an informal structure. It is crucial to recognize the makeup and the effects of both types of structures, or designs, in order to comprehend fully the ways in which the organization operates. In a highly complex organization, such as a hospital or other health care agency, the formal and informal structures are multiple, interrelated, overlapping, and simultaneous, so that careful observation and analysis are required to identify the various pathways for communication and decision making.

Formal structural designs are those designs that, on paper, feature clear-cut written and diagrammed policies, procedures, and detailed descriptions of job functions for employees at all levels of authority. The most traditional formal structure is a hierarchy, which may be represented as a pyramid, with a large number of relatively powerless people at the bottom and fewer, more powerful people in successively higher levels until the apex of the triangle is reached. Also known as the bureaucratic model, this structure is most readily apparent in the rank system of the military services. In health care, it is an outgrowth of the effects of military tradition on the care of the sick in the Middle Ages. With the advent of the Industrial Revolution, some minor changes were adopted to increase the efficiency of operating the institutions, but the basic organizational structure remained unchanged.

Within this traditional structure, subgroups are composed of people with similar backgrounds and special skills — for example, physicians in obstetrics, psychiatry, or pediatrics; nurses in oncology, medicine, or surgery; x-ray personnel; and dietary personnel. Such subgroupings and specialty areas lead to a cohesiveness within subgroups that serves to maintain the autonomy of each group. Although this unity can establish and maintain high morale among the group members, it can also make it difficult for group members to see beyond their own areas of interest. The group's energy is often spent in protecting itself rather than in furthering the goals of the organization. When there is a meeting between subgroups, problems can arise if each group works to maintain its own territorial rights rather than to approach the issue from a nonpartisan point of view.

The formal pyramid structure involves increasingly more specific responsibilities from top to bottom. In other words, the people at the top of the structure have general responsibilities for the organization as a whole, whereas personnel at the lower levels are more responsible for specific tasks within more narrowly defined areas. Also, each person is accountable not only for his own work but also for the work of all those below him in the hierarchy, just as each person must answer to others above him in the line of authority. These relationships, if viewed and implemented cooperatively, are quite constructive in meeting the short-term and long-term organizational objectives. Conflicts arise when superiors, subordinates, or both indulge in irresponsible behavior merely to demonstrate or resist authority per se.

Another formal design, which provides an alternative to the traditional hierarchical structure, is the matrix. The matrix structure provides a way of dealing with issues by means of groups that are formed to meet specific needs as they arise. A matrix is a collection of small suborganizations grouped together within the larger organizational design. Instead of depending on a flow of communication and decisions from one level of authority up or down to the next, as in a pyramid approach, personnel in a matrix are arranged according to particular functions, which they carry out with more autonomy than in a bureaucratic setting. Personnel communicate in any direction to obtain the assistance they need from other people or departments in fulfilling their particular functions. Negotiation, rather than issuing and obeying commands, becomes the major means of accomplishing the work objectives within a matrix design. Depending on the size and complexity of the agency, the structure may be strictly matrix or, as in most cases, a more traditional hierarchical structure that uses a matrix approach at or between various levels of authority.

Why did the matrix alternative arise with the health care delivery system? Until recent years, there seemed to be little opposition to the traditional bureaucratic format. Then, a reexamination of the organizational structure of health care institutions was necessitated by two major factors: the overwhelming complexity of the health care delivery system, brought about by rapidly advancing technology, and societal changes that have taken place in the postindustrial era.

A quick look at the modern hospital, whether it is a large medical center or a small community institution, will illustrate the complexity of modern health care delivery. The rapid expansion in medical technology has brought about means of caring for people that were undreamed of 50, or even 20, years ago. Monitoring systems, organ transplants, new diagnostic tests, "miracle" drugs, and other highly sophisticated materials and techniques have resulted in the proliferation of specialty groups and subgroups. Today, because of advanced medical and surgical technology and also because of basic population growth, patients in acute care facilities are greater in number and often more acutely ill than their predecessors, producing a dramatic impact on the quality and accessibility of health care services. On the other hand, many patients who in the past were hospitalized, notably ill children and patients of all ages who are chronically or terminally ill, now receive care in community settings rather than in the hospital. One result of these trends is the emergence of larger numbers of increasingly specialized professional and paraprofessional health care workers. In addition, the high cost of health care, the health insurance industry, and state and federal health care legislation are also influenced directly and indirectly by the boom in technology. In this kind of situation, people are less likely to be willing or even able to function at an optimal level within a rigidly structured, chain-of-command hierarchy. Instead, more opportunities are needed for free exchange of professional opinions from a variety of sources and across territorial lines within the organization.

The second factor, that of societal changes, is much more subtle and thus is frequently overlooked until one is forced by crisis to examine its impact. Recently in the United States, society has been moving from a position of emphasis on individual competition, independence, self-control, and high achievement, where great value was given to following orders efficiently and staying in line, to self-actualization, seeking happiness, and working cooperatively with others, where people want to participate meaningfully in making decisions that affect their life experiences. With these two factors at work, the strictly traditional organizational structure, which is fundamentally autocratic in nature, may not be the most efficient way to organize an agency.

The matrix approach, especially when combined with the traditional structure, gives an organization greater flexibility. This approach has other advantages in that it also helps to break down stereotypes and to foster collegiality within and between levels, further improving the quality of patient care.

A small institution, such as a community nursing agency, may have a pyramid structure on paper but function well with a semimatrix framework. The larger the agency, the more likely it is to follow the pyramid structure, although within that structure some departments may function with a matrix approach. Two examples of the matrix approach with a basic hierarchy are primary nursing and the multidisciplinary teams that are used in some hospital emergency rooms.

ORGANIZATIONAL DIAGRAM

Whatever its form, to be most functional, an organizational structure should be diagrammed and the diagram distributed and explained thoroughly to all employees. The organizational structure should be understood as more than just a chart illustrating lines of authority, division of labor, and channels of communication. Rather, it should be a frequently used tool for all employees in every area and at all levels of the organization. For example, within a hospital, the nursing department is responsible for coordinating many services that are required by patients. When problems arise, it is often the nurse who first learns about them, from the patient, the family, or another department. Frequently, an examination of the organizational chart can help to identify an effective solution to the problem and an idea of how to avoid the same problem in the future. Such an examination can also help to avoid one of the most common errors in initiating change, that of failing to make contact with representatives of all areas that may be affected, even slightly, by such a change. To assure reaching all employees (personnel, staff, etc.) concerned in solving a problem or initiating change to avoid certain problems, the organizational chart should be consulted at each step of the change process (see Chap. 7 for more detail).

The individual nurse should always consult the organizational chart in order to negotiate the system with an idea, problem, or question. Planning the most appropriate route to take can prevent a great deal of frustration, damaged self-confidence, and wasted time.

During preemployment interviews, nurses should always raise questions about the formal structure, ask to see the organizational chart, and note the various groups identified and the types of relationships delineated. It is important for a prospective employee to ask how strictly the formal channels of communication are adhered to, so that she can make a more informed decision about assuming a satisfying role within the organization. Also, are there interdepartmental ad hoc groups to discuss and settle issues? How do nurses and other employees at each level of authority contribute to the decision-making process?

When new or unfamiliar nursing positions are established, it is important not only for the administration to understand the relationships of these new positions to the already established positions but also for each member of the nursing staff to see clearly how she relates to the new positions within the context of the official organizational structure. A decade ago the importance of this process was clearly and somewhat uncomfortably underlined when the physician's assistant (PA) was introduced into the health care team. Although members of this group are legally accountable to the physicians, many nurses found themselves expected to accept responsibility for PAs in some aspects of their duties. Nurses who were well aware of the officially established lines of authority were best able to counteract and refuse this additional encroachment on their time and tasks, because they had a solid base from which to defend their point of view.

Another useful function of the organizational chart is the development of innovative organizational designs within the nursing department, which should be started only after examining what works and what does not work in the present structure. For example, when considering the substitution of a matrix pattern, such as primary nursing, for a hierarchical pattern, such as team nursing, a check of the organizational diagram should ensure that all appropriate groups and individuals are represented in considering the issues involved.

To be most useful, an organizational diagram should also indicate other types of relationships commonly found in service institutions. These relationships may involve individuals or groups outside the employ of the agency. The most common types are contractual, cooperative, coordinating, and advisory relationships.

The affiliation of a school of nursing with a hospital or community nursing agency demonstrates two such relationships. The contractual relationship is between the administration of the educational institution and the nursing service administration of the health care delivery agency; it delineates the roles of students, faculty, and hospital staff in the clinical area. The cooperative relationship refers to different individuals or groups working together for a common purpose and is well illustrated by the planning carried out by the clinical instructor, head nurse, and nursing staff as they cooperate to meet the ultimate goal of quality patient care.

A coordinating relationship is a somewhat less formal, harmonious, voluntary combination that occurs, more or less spontaneously, between two or more individuals or groups who have no official relationship. The advisory type of relationship is a more recent, frequent occurrence, particularly when federal funds are involved in a health care project. Legal guidelines established by the legislature for such projects frequently stipulate that consumer advisory groups must be involved. The purpose of an advisory relationship is for the advisory group to make recommendations and offer suggestions, on the basis of an underlying belief that such assistance will be given full consideration by the organization. An even more common advisory relationship is that between the director of nursing and the board of directors of the agency.

INFORMAL ORGANIZATIONAL STRUCTURE

In addition to a formal structure, every organization also has an informal structure. In many instances, the informal structure is the actual working structure, so a careful investigation of the informal structure is always essential for understanding accurately what is really going on within the organization.

The very formal structure that was developed for efficiency can also be manipulated by clever individuals to stymie change. The red tape and waiting periods inherent in extremely complex institutions can become unbearably frustrating for each employee. Therefore, all organizations gradually develop informal means to avoid some of the red tape and to implement needed changes, while still working within the official system.

The degree to which the informal structure is actually defined, either orally or in writing, varies from institution to institution. However, in most cases the informal structure is not documented in writing, so the best method of discovering it is by direct observation of the unofficial relationships and communication channels in which employees at all levels are active. An investigator of the informal structure phenomenon is always careful to keep her eyes and ears open, constantly reminding herself of the following types of guidelines:

- Who sits with whom at meals and coffee breaks, day after day? Observe with whom people choose to sit at meetings and staff development programs.
- Which people carpool together, socialize together? Listen for people who continually support or oppose one another on issues.
- Which subgroups interact with ease?
- Which subgroups avoid one another?
- Who always supports new ideas?
- Who always criticizes new ideas?
- Who neither supports new ideas nor offers constructive criticism?
- Who speaks out in the various subgroups?
- Who listens?

Such observations will assist in identifying the informal organizational structure, through which much useful work can be accomplished. When appointing ad hoc groups, the wise leader uses key people within the informal structure rather than limiting the choice to officially designated leaders, in order to assure the greatest success.

Staff nurses sometimes feel overwhelmed when first confronted with the challenge of analyzing and influencing the organizational structure of their work situation. As a result, sometimes they merely settle for a passive role in which crucial organizational decisions are made without their active participation.

However, if nurses at all levels of authority make a definitive effort to understand the formal and informal structure and to maintain a strong voice in how the institution is run, they can exert enormous influence on the organizational goals, structure, policies, activities, and other characteristics of the working environment. Nurses who take the time to familiarize themselves with the map of the health care institution in which they practice are far more likely to be able to function effectively than their colleagues whose vision is strictly limited by their immediate surroundings.

BIBLIOGRAPHY

Periodicals

Abalos DT: Strategies of transformation in the health delivery system. *Nurs Forum* 17:284–316, 1978.

Brown BJ, et al: Affecting nursing goals in health care. *Nurs Adm Q* 2:17–31, Spring 1978.

Clark C: Learning to negotiate the system. *Nurs Outlook* 25:39, January 1977.

Cutler MJ: Nursing leadership and management: an historical perspective. *Nurs Adm Q* 1:7–19, Fall 1976.

Kalisch BJ: The promise of power. *Nurs Outlook* 26:42–46, January 1978.

Schuldt S: Supervision and the informal organization. *J Nurs Adm* 8:21–25, July 1978.

Books

Albanese R: *Management: Toward Accountability of Performance.* Homewood, Ill, Richard D. Irwin Inc, 1975.

Bentley P: *Health Care Agencies and Professionals: A Changing Relationship,* National League for Nursing, Publication 14–1669. New York, 1977, pp. 1–8.

Beyers M, Phillips C: *Nursing Management for Patient Care,* ed 2. Boston, Little Brown & Co, 1979.

Brooten DA, et al: *Leadership for Change: A Guide for the Frustrated Nurse.* Philadelphia, JB Lippincott Co, 1978.

Yura H, Ozimek D, Walsh MB: *Nursing Leadership: Theory and Process.* New York, Appleton-Century-Crofts, 1976.

3. Quality Assurance and Accountability in Health Care Delivery

"Cope With or Cop Out"

Joyce L. Schweiger, R.N., M.S.

BEHAVIORAL OBJECTIVES

After reviewing this chapter, the reader will be able to

- list the major factors described that have had a direct effect on quality assurance within the health care system
- identify those areas where nursing care would be effective in assuring quality care and increasing accountability in health care settings
- compare and contrast specifically described methods used to evaluate the quality of care provided
- identify the impetus the federal government has had in establishing programs to ensure quality care in health care agencies
- identify who is accountable for the care provided to the patient in relation to areas of clinical specialization

Quality assurance may be defined as a measure of competence demonstrated by efficiency in performance. It also includes evaluation of process (operational activities related to nursing) and evaluation of the outcome of process based on meeting the patient's individual needs in accordance with predetermined standards set by the agency and those standards expected by the patient and his significant others.

Assurance is not a new concept, having been defined in general terms in the past. Today, the definition has become more explicit with specific reference to accountability in the provision of quality care. Words and documentation alone are not sufficient evidence to justify actions in providing quality care today. The demand is for measurable methods to support documentation. In the past, nurses have considered themselves accountable but within certain limits.

Accountability was and still is frequently confused with responsibility. Kron defines both terms clearly: *responsibility* refers to what should be done, the expected action; *accountability* is concerned with what was done as compared with what should have been done (1). Many nurses, without realizing it, have been more responsible than accountable for their actions. They have identified what they perceived as the patient's needs and have tried to meet them. Many times they have done this without questioning which needs the patient, or his significant others, felt had higher priority.

There is no doubt that patient welfare has been a specific concern of health care providers since the middle of the nineteenth century. This concern for patient welfare had been identified by Florence Nightingale in 1853 (2), but again it was presented in the context of responsible action, not accountable action.

One of the early organized attempts to ensure excellence in hospital care was undertaken with the founding of the American College of Surgeons in 1913, from which grew the Joint Commission on Accreditation for Hospitals (JCAH). However, the JCAH initially lacked nurse representation. The Joint Commission now involves nurses in determining standards of practice and in participation on evaluation teams. It has also expanded to explore its standards for quality and quality assurance in other health care settings (2, p. 34). In addition, the federal government has passed legislation that has provided specific direction for the provision of quality care. One of the most effective of these measures to monitor the patient's welfare and health care is contained in the Amendment to the Social Security Act of 1972, Public Law 92-603 (3). This amendment states, in part, that Professional Standards Review Organizations (PSRO) are responsible for reviewing all institutional services and the practices of *all* professionals delivering these services. The legislation is directed toward quality assurance and accountability and has provided momentum to those concerned members of the profession who have desired to participate effectively in providing quality patient care.

Within the past decade, quality care has become not only a professional concern but a public demand. The public has been disillusioned for a long time with the health care delivery system. Public protest over cost and quality of care has forced health care professionals to pull back sharply and in some instances, defensively to reassess and reevaluate the system's approach to the delivery of care.

FACTORS AFFECTING QUALITY HEALTH CARE

Four major factors have probably had the greatest impact on the thinking of health care providers and have directly affected quality care within the health care system: cost, consumerism, organizational complexity, and care sharing. Each factor must be carefully examined in order to understand their collective effect.

Cost

Health care is now more costly than national defense. The causes for this increase in spending have been attributed to population growth, an increase in both the use and intensity of health care service, price inflation, and duplication of service. In the two decades between World War II and the advent of the Medicare and Medicaid programs, 21% of the increase in national health costs was attributed to a growth in population. After 1965, the rate of population increase lessened and, by 1975, this decline in growth rate accounted for only a 6% rise in health care cost (4). Since 1975, cost increases have been attributed directly to advances in technology, along with an increase in cost for specialized services that include highly trained personnel. An additional cost increase that has been overlooked frequently is product price inflations.

Cost factors for hospital items from various departments are listed in Table 3-1. The data are self-explanatory and substantiate the need for health care facilities frequently to raise the cost of bed and board to the consumer. However, the consumer should be made aware of what he is paying for and why he is paying. This major factor is frequently overlooked when it is necessary to raise the price of bed and board per diem in health care agencies. Many inquiries about such increases are made by consumers who are not aware of the hidden costs. Seeing a large increase in salary budget allocations, consumers tend to attribute the increased expenses only to salaries. Such a conclusion is not

Table 3-1. Escalation of Selected Hospital Costs, 1974–1979

	1974	1979	% Increase
X-ray film			
14 x 17 Dupont Cronex 4; 500 sheets	$348.20	$485.70	39%
Cost per sheet	.6964	.9714	
Drugs			
Triavil 2-25 tablet, 100 units	10.30	13.76	34%
Cost per unit	.103	.138	
Gowns			
Barrier surgical gown, small;			
case of 32 gowns	46.60	85.42	83%
Cost per gown	1.456	2.669	
IV solutions			
5% Dextrose + 0.9% Sod. 500 ml	7.568	14.021	85%
Natural gas			
Per 100 cu ft	.1018	.2841	179%
Fuel oil, gal	.2990	.594	99%
Food: Top round beef, per lb	1.36	1.93	42%

Permission for publication of data granted by Community General Hospital, Reading, Pa., June 1979.

unexpected, since the consumer is rarely made aware of the inflation in cost purchases of products and hospital uses.

Price inflation is apparent in other ways. For example, health care insurance has added to the increase in cost because the insurance plans generally favor hospitalization rather than ambulatory care services. Unfortunately, health care insurance does not cover all costs associated with medical care (5). Therefore, the expense to the consumer is compounded.

Price inflation becomes a vicious cycle when services are duplicated. For example, three hospitals in a region may be interested in purchasing their own CAT scanner, the super-fast, three-dimensional x-ray machine. The machine costs more than $500,000. Other hospitals in the same region have scanners that are available to the hospitals that wish to purchase the equipment. The area's health planning organization has investigated the requests and has determined that the purchases are not needed. The hospitals in turn may choose to ignore the regional planning organizations' advice and purchase the scanners. What is the result? The hospitals involved could lose state and federal reimbursment through Medicare and Medicaid for interest on and depreciation of the equipment. There may also be a possibility that Blue Cross may cut off service payments to the patient for the scanners, even though the scanner is a very valuable diagnostic tool. As a result, health care costs to the consumers are inflated.

The areas mentioned reflect the spending cost to the consumer. They also identify a glaring absence of accountability on the part of the health care providers. It is apparent that vested interests are not in the best interest of the consumer.

Consumerism

The second factor, consumerism, is equally as forceful an impact as cost. Consumerism includes the patient's need for recognition as a member of the health care team. It is imperative that the patients be permitted to exercise their right to participate in making those decisions that they believe will ultimately affect their care. Their need to become actively involved in their health care has been fostered by

1. dissatisfaction with care received in health care agencies
2. increase in cost for care delivery as previously discussed
3. expanded information about health care via public media and the lay literature

For example, in a nursing journal article (6), a consumer spoke about the care-related deficiencies he encountered, starting with preadmission and proceeding through his hospitalization to his discharge. Many of the situations he described would be familiar to us. It is because of such personal experiences and media publicity that patients are demanding a voice in the way health care is delivered and financed. They want to be active participants on governing and advisory boards. They want to be certain that the Patients' Bill of Rights does not become merely words on a plaque in a hospital lobby or a typed paper given to patients in the admission office. Patients want to be certain that they receive what they are promised, and they believe this can be achieved by their active participation. This demand by the silent majority must now be recognized, accepted, and responded to by health care providers.

Organization Complexity

The third factor affecting the health care delivery system is agency organization and bureaucratic complexity. The complexity of the agencies involves not only an external expanse in size and structure but also the internal multifaceted bureaucratic structure, the agency administration. Decisions are no longer totally in the hands of the selected board of governors. The bureaucracy has become more complex. Decisions and recommendations come from advisory boards and committees that are composed of representatives from all departments within the agency, as well as from outside representatives that may have subcontracts with the agency.

Outside pressure from the state and federal government have also affected this decision-making process. For example, the safety committee within the hospital is made up of many department representatives, but their decisions are controlled on a federal level by the Occupational Safety and Health Act (OSHA, Public Law 91-596, passed in 1970). Any change they may decide on must be within the regulations of OSHA before decisions can be implemented.

In addition, the concepts of the administrative structure for decision making are changing. Concepts of hierarchical organization other

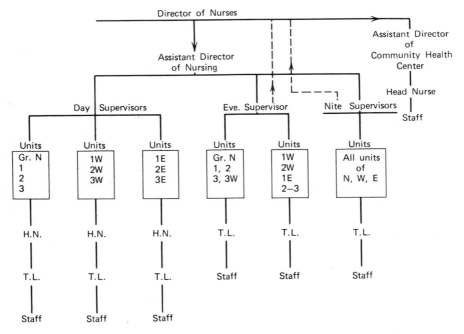

Figure 3-1. A pyramid nursing service structure that shows centralization of power with several levels of hierarchy. Basic premise of this organizational structure is title and rank. Work distribution is determined by size and number of clinical areas rather than by consideration for areas of specialization with representation of expertise.

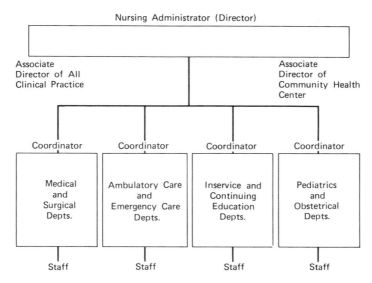

Figure 3-2. A flat nursing service structure that shows decentralization of power, few levels of authority distribution. Basic premise is to emphasize coordination of activities, strengthen professional nursing practice, and provide opportunities for specialization by prepared practitioners.

than the traditional tall structure are being used. The prevailing idea has been that an organization is only as effective as its basic structure, and that an effective structure reaps the advantages of specialization, technology, and division of work. With this in mind, many agencies have now introduced the flat organization structure concept. This concept allows both horizontal and vertical dimensions, permitting a larger span of control (4, pp. 171–172) (see Figs. 3-1 and 3-2).

Centralization, alone or in conjunction with decentralization, is another important concept. Centralization keeps decision making in the hands of a few, with little regard for input from the majority. The emphasis is on the degree of differences involved in delegation of responsibilities of power and authority through the chain of command. Decentralization, however, lends itself to individual accountability. It allows for a free flow of ideas and information. For example, in nursing, decentralization in relation to standards of patient care and nursing practice allows the nursing staff to have a part in the decision-making process. Staff input will be received and reviewed by nursing administration. This will not free the nursing administrator from the responsibility and the authority for final decision making, but it will enhance the staff's awareness of their role as decision makers and planners. Decentralization stresses and reemphasizes the nurse's accountability in the provision of quality care. This is particularly true when the ideas, suggestions, or changes the staff have recommended are accepted as policy, procedure, or changes in standards of practice. Sharing the power for decision making can only eventually strengthen the efforts of the health care professional in providing quality care.

Care Sharing

The fourth factor that has forced recognition of the importance of quality in health care delivery is care sharing. There are professionals within the health care system who believe that fragmentation of care will always exist among care providers and that there is little need to expect change. This reasoning is based on individual insecurity. It reflects a reluctance on the part of care providers to recognize and accept specialized and diversified preparation among their professional colleagues. They are hesitant to share patient care with the people who can supply the expertise necessary to assume that the patient is receiving quality care. In spite of this reaction, the demand for accountability in patient care is forcing the providers to accept care sharing.

The professional nurse can no longer be the catchall for left-over activities. The potential of each person on the health care team must be used to its maximum. Whoever is qualified to tell the patient how to put the hospital care plan into effect at home will do so. Whoever is best qualified to explain to the patient why medications are ordered and what result will be expected from the medication will do so. Whoever is best qualified to develop a plan of respiratory care of physical therapy for the patient/client will do so. Whoever is best qualified to explain to the patient and his family the nutritional values of a specific diet will do so. In each case, the information will be shared with all the health care team members. This is care sharing, not fragmentation. Fragmentation occurs when communication ceases among those involved in providing care.

The four factors — cost, consumerism, organization complexity, and care sharing — have had and will continue to have the greatest collective effect on the delivery of health care and must be recognized and dealt with objectively rather than overlooked.

ROLE OF NURSING IN THE HEALTH CARE SYSTEM

As a major subsystem of the larger health care system, nursing must be more explicit in its specific role in fostering quality assurance in patient care. The tools available to nurses to measure quality care must now be put into practice selectively. This is the responsibility of decision makers at every level of health care delivery. The most practical and available tools are sometimes the ones nurses overlook or tend to take for granted.

Nursing staff can measure quality care by using any or all of the following methods: nursing rounds, peer review, patient questionnaires, audit, patient consumer advocate, and professional role expansion. If the nursing department does not concern itself with such measurement, a lack of concern for patient welfare is indicated. At one time it was permissible to claim ignorance regarding the implementation of methods to measure quality care, but with today's resources this is no longer feasible. Each method will not only measure the quality care provided but reflect accountability in a variety of ways. The methods deserve individual attention in order to distinguish the effectiveness of each.

Nursing Rounds

Agencies that have nursing rounds use them in different ways—as a system of reporting from shift to shift, as teaching rounds for staff, as a part of evaluation of staff performance, and in determining patient categorization for care assignments. Each use ultimately is valuable in determining the quality of patient care.

Reporting rounds provide the nurses with informative data about the patients they are visiting. Rounds allow the nurses to associate the problems and needs of a specific patient with an identity, a face, and a name, not just a diagnosis and a number. As a reporting tool, rounds give the reporting nurse an opportunity to rethink the data presented and perhaps add to them while conferring with the patient or family. Rounds will phase out uninformative reports, such as "the same," "no change," or "slept all night." Rounds avoid personal opinions and expressions of feelings related to a specific patient that do not belong in a report but would be better said or discussed in care conferences.

As a teaching aid nursing rounds add another dimension. Teaching rounds are an excellent way to evaluate the patient, both physically and psychosocially. The rounds provide an opportunity to assess the patient and to compare and substantiate findings with chart data to determine the degree of improvement or change. The patient, as well as his environment, is evaluated at this time. This evaluation may provide additional information about the patient that can be incorporated into his plan of care. It also provides an opportunity to communicate with the patient on an individual basis. Ordinarily, both communication and evaluation may not occur during the scheduled activities of the day except to staff specifically assigned to provide his care. Teaching rounds naturally lend themselves to observation and evaluation of the care provider's performance.

The quality of care given by either a group or one practitioner can be evaluated by supervisors and peers. Evaluation allows the practitioner the opportunity to ask questions and provide information about each patient. At the same time, it will allow the evaluator the opportunity to identify the strengths and weaknesses of the practitioner, determine the patient's satisfaction with his care, and observe the organizational capabilities of the participants. Rounds used in this context, however, must be frequent and not just before an evaluation period, or they may lose their effectiveness.

Categorizing patients in order to determine the distribution of a patient work load makes it necessary for those assigning the care to go beyond the chart or Kardex to determine patient priorities. Patients must be seen, and nursing rounds provide a good opportunity for this. A patient may need little physical care but a great deal of psychosocial support that can be time consuming, but this too must be considered. Rounds will aid the unit leader in gathering data to determine the daily staffing pattern needed, as well as to plan long-range care. Nursing rounds alone will not assure quality patient care, but they are a major step in that direction if used appropriately and the resulting information applied to practice.

Peer Review

In 1977, a survey questionnaire was distributed by Brooten et al (2, pp. 146–147). Of the 362 nurses who responded, 177 were in practice settings, and 185 were in education settings. The survey clearly showed that peer review was one of the priority mechanisms nurses felt should be used to ensure quality patient care; 77% of all respondents attested to this. Peer review was surpassed only by outcome criteria (goals for patient care), which received 80%. The survey also showed that 52% of all of the participants believed a review of performance of nurses should be done by those nurses working at the peer level who are informed of the criteria for peer review. These data are strong indicators that peer review is an essential item as a supportive mechanism for quality assurance and accountability in patient care and should be a priority to consider for agency use.

Patient Questionnaires

Questionnaires should be developed as quality assurance tools. If questionnaires are well constructed, measurable, and not ambiguous, they can provide direct input from the patient about the care he received. This information is difficult to obtain by any other means. Questionnaires can be given to the patient while he is still in the agency (concurrent) or after he has been discharged (retrospective). Either way, the staff has an opportunity for feedback. A problem that may occur with the questionnaire, if given to the patient while hospitalized, is that the result may have a halo effect—that is, the patient who is hospitalized may tend to give a glowing report that, in some instances, could be unreliable. On the other hand, if the questionnaire is sent to the patient's home, the bias may be in the opposite direction—based upon one unpleasant experience. For this reason, it is wise to employ additional methods in order to measure accurately the degree of competence in performance that exists in your facility.

Nursing Audit

Space does not permit enough content here, particularly if staff are unfamiliar with or presently struggling with the audit process. Audit is now considered mandatory by JCAH standards and is included as a part of federal regulations.

Audit is the measure of care received by the patient after a cycle of care has been completed. This can be carried out before or after the patient is discharged. Audit involves the examination of the patient's chart by qualified practitioners who have developed care criteria to measure the level of performance. Criteria are based upon the department's philosophy, standards of performance, and goals.

The audit provides specific data for the supervisors/head nurses in regard to

• areas of needed patient care improvement

- basis for inservice education
- need for teaching/supervision
- individual staff members who give direct patient care (7)

The audit also supplies information for head nurses and staff about

- self-examination of care in their specific nursing unit or setting
- identification of types of care in which improvement will depend on the staff acquisition of additional knowledge or skills (7)

Nursing audits may be as complex or as simple as the agency feels is required. In all instances, audits must reflect the quality of care provided.

Patient/Consumer Advocate

Advocacy is not a new concept in nursing, but it has not received the recognition it deserves. Now it is more open and direct, a role that can be assigned to one nurse or considered as a part of the role of all who participate in patient care. Either way, the role of advocate should be an accepted responsibility for members of the health care team. The patient advocate does not merely make the patient aware of his rights; if the patient is unable to exercise those rights, the patient advocate provides necessary assistance. The patient advocate is accountable for the care provided to the patient and, therefore, should have access to all the patient's hospital records, the ability to call in qualified consultants, the opportunity and responsibility to participate in hospital committees monitoring patient care, the right and ability to lodge complaints directly to hospital administration, ability to delay discharges and to participate at the patient's request and direction in discussing his case (5, p. 59).

The patient advocate role is one that can cause turbulence, particularly for care providers who do not willingly accept criticism or who are threatened by the possibility that the care they have given the patients may be less than optimum. This is not a valid reason for avoiding the issue. Personal reactions are not the concern; the patient is. If patient advocate is an assigned role in a hospital setting, it should be assigned to a professional nurse, not a social worker, psychologist, or lay person. The nurse's preparations in meeting both the physical and psychosocial needs of the patient and her knowledge of the agency structure make her a preferred choice. In any health care agency, the patient advocate should be the most qualified professional on the staff who has access to all departments and areas within the agency and reports directly to the agency top administration. The person who is assigned the role must have good rapport with the other health professionals on the team so that intervention is feasible. Of all the tools suggested to aid in the improvement of quality care, the patient advocate role is probably the most difficult to fulfill, but it is one of the most valuable.

Role Expansion

Role expansion can be used to enhance quality patient care. The nurse's role can extend across and beyond the lines of many established health care systems. Nurses can be found in a variety of roles that include family nurse clinicians, pediatric nurse practitioners, nurse midwives, independent practitioners, and primary nurses. In each role, the nurse has an opportunity to evaluate, to enhance, and to ensure the provision of quality care through her own intervention and accountability for the care she provides either directly or indirectly.

With the increased expansion of roles in specialized fields of patient care and with the nurse as a primary provider of care, we can demonstrate improvement in care to the patient. However, in order to use effectively even one of the suggested methods to measure performance, the nursing staff as a whole must be involved. Needs for change should not have to be identified by the agency hierarchy alone. Methods of performance should not have to be dictated by the agency hierarchy alone. Both areas should be recognized as a responsibility of *all* participants in patient care, both up the line as well as down. When this occurs in nursing, one of the major subsystems in the health care system, an important step will have been taken to make accountability a reality in the quality assurance process.

REFERENCES

1. Kron T: *The Management of Patient Care,* ed 4. Philadelphia, WB Saunders Co, 1976, p. 25.
2. Brooten D, et al: *Leadership for Change: A Guide for the Frustrated Nurse.* New York, JB Lippincott Co, 1978, p. 33.
3. Public Law 92-603, 92nd Congress HRI, Oct. 30, 1972, pp. 101–117.
4. Alexander E: *Nursing Administration in the Hospital Health Care System,* ed 2. St Louis, The CV Mosby Co, 1978, p. 17.
5. Davis AJ, Aroskar M: *Ethical Dilemmas and Nursing Practice.* New York, Appleton-Century-Crofts, 1978, p. 59.

6. A consumer speaks out about hospital care. *Am J Nurs* 76:1443, September 1976.
7. Stone S, et al: *Management for Nurses*. St Louis, The CV Mosby Co, 1976, p. 230.

BIBLIOGRAPHY

Periodicals

Annas GJ, Healey J: The patient rights advocate. *J Nurs Adm* 4:25–31, May-June 1974.
Besch LB: Informed consent: a patient's right. *Nurs Outlook* 27:32, January 1979.
Block D: Evaluation of nursing care in term of process and outcome: issues in research and quality assurance. *Nurs Digest* 6:32–41, Winter 1979.
Brown BJ (ed): Quality assurance and peer review. *Nurs Adm Q* 1: Spring 1977.
Fifer WR: Quality assurance: debate persists on goals, impact, and methods of evaluating case. *Hospitals* 53:163, April 1, 1979.
Hoover J, et al: Nursing quality assurance: the Wisconsin system. *Nurs Outlook* 26:242, April 1978.
Moore KR: What nurses learn from nursing audit. *Nurs Outlook* 27:254, April 1979.
Schmadl JC: Quality assurance: examination of the concept. *Nurs Outlook* 27:462, July 1979.

Books

Alexander EL: *Nursing Administration in the Health Care System,* ed 2. St Louis, The CV Mosby Co, 1978.
Brooten D, et al: *Leadership for Change: A Guide for the Frustrated Nurse.* Philadelphia, JB Lippincott Co, 1978.
Davis AJ, Aroskar MA: *Ethical Dilemmas and Nursing Practice.* New York, Appleton-Century-Crofts, 1978.
Kron T: *The Management of Patient Care,* ed 4. Philadelphia, WB Saunders Co, 1976.
McCool B, Brown M: *The Management Response: Conceptual, Technical and Human Skills of Health Administration.* Philadelphia, WB Saunders Co, 1977.
Mayers MG, et al: *Quality Assurance for Patient Care.* New York, Appleton-Century-Crofts, 1977.
Stone S, et al (eds): *Management for Nurses: A Multidisciplinary Approach.* St Louis, The CV Mosby Co, 1976.

4. Leadership Styles

"Be a Leader, Not a Boss"

Joyce L. Schweiger, R.N., M.S.,
and Mary Lou Hamilton, R.N., M.S.

BEHAVIORAL OBJECTIVES

After reviewing this chapter, the reader will be able to

- identify the relationship between leadership and management
- identify two levels of leadership
- list situations in which leadership styles can adapt to change
- identify the nurse's own predominant leadership style and those of her coworkers
- compare and contrast the basic styles of leadership
- select the appropriate leadership style to bring about change in her particular health care agency

No matter what her title or position, the professional nurse must accept responsibility and accountability for her leadership role in health care delivery. To do this effectively, she must have an understanding of leadership styles, both her own and those with which she interacts. For example, the new graduate in her first position may find herself in the role of delegating responsibility to members of her team, leading small groups, and presiding at conferences. Each role requires her to give direction to or to manage people. Her leadership style will be the key factor in the effectiveness of her management.

In order to become a recognized leader of nursing personnel, it is important not only to understand one's own dominant leadership style but to understand the styles of others. The basic leadership style of supervisors is not likely to change, even with much training and experience. However, if a nurse is aware of a person's leadership style, then she is able to work more effectively to attain specific goals. The situation in which the staff nurse has a good idea but does not act on it because she believes it will get nowhere coming from her is not uncommon. Nevertheless, if she knows the leadership styles of those who will act on her suggestions, she can present her ideas and plans in a way that would be most acceptable to her leader. This is a form of manipulating the behavior of others.

LEADERSHIP AND MANAGEMENT

Leadership and *management* are two terms used that need further clarification. Although the terms are frequently used interchangeably, Yura, Ozimek, and Walsh (1, p. 121) have made an interesting distinction between them: leaders may use principles of management and supervision, but not all administrators, managers, and supervisors are leaders. A review of the literature indicates that numerous periodicals and books explain and define leadership and management in industrial, medical, and nursing settings. Despite all these sources, there are still questions about what makes an effective leader.

Personal traits have been described to indicate what mades a good leader, but recently this has been considered misdirected information to a certain extent. Merton refutes the premise that distinctive traits of leaders provide an understanding of leadership. He suggests that leadership is derived from another perspective other than individual traits of leaders. This perspective, he says, "involves attributes of the transactions between those who lead and those who follow" (2). Therefore, leadership approached with this perspective in mind would be the result of a compatible interaction among people.

Nursing leadership is defined by Stevens "as the ability of the nurse managers to convince other unit personnel to work toward the attainment of the organization, unit, and patient care objectives" (3).

It is the nurse-manager who provides the primary unifying force that will bring people in a nursing unit together to work effectively to achieve mutual goals. In order to do this, motivational techniques are employed (see Chap. 8). Leadership is seen as a unifying, motivating force that creates a fertile environment in which a nursing staff becomes productive in achieving quality patient care goals and also in fulfilling staff needs.

Management is similar to leadership in meaning. It is a dimension described by Yura, Ozimek, and Walsh (1, p. 122) as a method by which goals are reached. Management is defined as the "conduct or direction of anything, including wielding, controlling, dealing, carrying on and handling" (4). Management means "control of the process of executing given policy and is clearly distinguished from the formulation and determination of policy and the activities involved and abilities required, which are seen as administration" (5, p. 252). Tannenbaum and others (5, p. 263) state that a person is a manager and manages only if she has and uses formal authority to direct, organize, or control responsible subordinates. She is a nonmanager unless conformity to these specifications occurs. Leadership becomes an integral part of the management process.

Manipulation

The relationship between leadership and management can be seen more readily when a third dimension is introduced — *manipulation,* defined by Webster in 1970 (6) as "skillful handling or operation, artful management or control. . . ." This being the case, leadership is essentially the art of effective manipulation, and leadership style is how one goes about manipulating persons and things to accomplish a goal. Manipulation can carry a positive connotation where it becomes a technique of management that accomplishes patient care objectives through the actions of others.

LEVELS OF LEADERSHIP

With these definitions, leaders may be identified at all levels of the health care team, which raises another aspect — leadership on two levels, formal and informal. Formal leadership is leadership with authority, and informal leadership is leadership without designated authority. The latter results from one's ability to lead, based upon personality, skill in interacting with others, and the wish to dominate. The leader is not formally appointed but is accepted by the members of the informal group (7). Although our main concern is leadership with authority, it is equally important to examine the situation arising from leadership without authority. It is in this situation that potential for formal leadership may be recognized in a person. It is also important to identify the informal leader, as she can be a key figure in implementing change and in motivating staff to accept change. According to Beach (8), the status of this informal leader may be derived in part from a position held in the formal organizational structure. This can be based on her past contribution to the group's purposes, exceptional skill, extensive knowledge of technology, or being especially helpful to associates. Recognizing this style and capitalizing upon it produce positive results. (This issue will be discussed further in Chaps. 7 and 8.)

An example of leadership without authority occurred with Team 1 on a surgical unit. The team leader was a new graduate who had been working on the unit for three months and was the designated leader with authority. When the team received reports from the night nurse, a member of the team who was a licensed practical nurse (LPM) asked many pertinent questions. At the end of the report, she asked the team leader about the assignment of nonpatient care tasks; before the LPN was given an answer, she had already worked out the details with the other team members. As a result, throughout the day the team members went to her with questions that did not pertain to patient care. Later in the day the LPN asked if the staff might hold a team conference about one of her patients, and they agreed. This was an LPN functioning as a leader without authority. In this situation, she was primarily a positive influence on the team. However, not all informal leadership is positive in nature. Almost everyone has been involved in a situation in which there is a strong informal leader in the group who presents a negative influence that blocks the informal group interaction and brings anger or frustration to the formal leader. To work with the informal leader and organization, the formal leader must accept certain facts: the informal leader and informal organization/group exist and have a profound effect upon people; and, although at times the effect may be diverse, the formal leader who recognizes and comprehends the group dynamics of the situation can maximize its potential value (9).

Leadership with authority does not necessarily mean successful leadership. According to Merton, "Authority involves the legitimated rights of a position that require others to obey; leadership is an interpersonal relation in which others comply because they want to, not because they have to" (2). Influence beyond the delegated authority does not depend solely on the personality of the leader involved and her leadership style but also on her awareness of the input importance and of combining leadership with authority. The appointed leader is not always the most popular person, whereas the informal leader is usually a popular person among her peers.

CHARACTERISTICS OF EFFECTIVE LEADERSHIP

Many studies have been carried out to determine the characteristics of an effective leader, and a long list has been compiled. However, it would seem that, since leadership involves a direct influence upon others and results in collective action, it would be better, as Merton says, "to seek its workings in the systems of roles and interaction between people rather than simply in the characteristics of individuals" (2).

The effective leader is able to accept both success and failure with grace. She is a risk taker, one who attempts new things with the realization that some efforts will be won and others lost (10). When faced with a defeat, she does not seek scapegoats to blame but accepts responsibility for her actions. It is equally important for the effective leader to accept success gracefully. The leader who dwells upon her successes soon becomes boring and less effective in her interpersonal relationships. The inability to accept success is not an unusual response in today's society. This attitude is probably a remnant of the Puritan ethic. An example is seen in the process of self-evaluation. Frequently those people who are rated highest by peers and superiors will rate themselves as average—or at least below others' evaluations of them. The successful leader is able to evaluate herself honestly and with an open mind.

The person in a leadership position is faced with many frustrations, but her effectiveness is influenced by how those frustrations are handled. If the leader displays frustration, the staff quickly responds in a similar manner. When dealing with frustration, such as defeat, hostile behavior may be evident. Hostile behavior is seen more frequently in the authoritarian type of leader. When her direction is not taken and defeat follows, angry defensive behavior is seen. The effect of her response on the group may be to take sides or join forces against the leader. In either case, this effect is disruptive to staff, other health care team members and, most important, to the patient and family, as the staff may become defensive with them.

Effective leaders have self-respect and are able to share themselves with others because of their self-assurance. They are interested in accomplishments and are often involved in several projects at one time. They also have a realistic picture of how far they can extend themselves.

Effective leaders have a special outlook on work. They are hard workers, but they do not interpret work as hard. They do not ask, "What is in it for me?" They do not intentionally seek external rewards. Their motivation is internal, obtaining satisfaction from a job well done. These leaders create a desirable environment and an attitude among their subordinates toward accomplishing the goals and objectives of their department, unit, or team (11). In nursing management, a person should become a manager because she enjoys this role, particularly since the role is frequently laden with frustrations.

EFFECTIVE APPROACHES TO PROBLEMS

There are typical ways in which effective leaders approach people and problems. A problem should be approached in terms of specific needs of people rather than in terms of the mechanics of the problem itself. For example: Mr. Adams was in the terminal stages of cancer. He and his wife had no children but did have a miniature poodle that was treated like a member of the family. Having been in the hospital for four months, Mr. Adams missed his dog and frequently asked about him. Arrangements were made to place Mr. Adams on a stretcher and take him to the ambulance entrance so he could see his dog. When the time came, it was clear that he was unable to travel the distance, and he became very depressed. The acting charge nurse for the weekend suggested that Mrs. Adams bring the dog to Mr. Adams. The staff will never forget the incident and the positive effect it had on Mr. Adams.

What kind of effect did this decision have on the staff and nursing administration? Two approaches to this situation are most common. The first would result in memos appearing the following day reminding the staff of the policy that under no circumstances are pets to be allowed in the hospital. This would be solving the problem through a mechanical approach but ignore the feelings of people involved. The second would be to discuss the situation with the staff working with the patient, taking into consideration the particulars of the situation and the thought processes that led to the staff's judgment to ignore policy. This would be approaching the problem in terms of the needs of people. The second approach was used in this incident. However, in each approach, a clue was given to the type of leadership involved.

LEADERSHIP STYLES

Three common leadership styles have been generally accepted: autocratic, democratic, and laissez-faire. The autocrat makes decisions alone and, although she may be essentially correct in her thinking, she lacks the supportive power that results in decisions made with consultation. At the other end of the continuum is the democratic leader, who allows freedom in discussion and input from subordinates that result in diffusion of decision making (12). There are degrees along the continuum that fall near either the autocratic or the democratic approach. Frequently the leadership style that is employed by the leader will often be dependent upon the particular situation or problem. The laissez-faire style is described as one that stays in the middle of the continuum, not moving in any particular direction or accomplishing anything of a constructive nature. It is at times a holding style of leadership, one that is frequently used when a nursing administration is undergoing a period of transition. For example, the nursing leader may have resigned her position and a temporary leader been appointed to fill the void until the permanent replacement has arrived or been selected. This temporary leader may have been told to "hold the fort," "keep things on an even keel" or "status quo," and make no changes. Depending upon the span of time between the appointed formal leaders, this situation can produce some unfortunate outcomes. It can result in a demoralizing effect upon staff and inadvertently effect the quality of patient care.

There are additional styles that are used in the clinical setting. Leininger (13) favors a confrontation-negotiation style of leadership as opposed to the earlier establishment-maintenance style. Today nurse administrations are expected to cope with complex management problems, critical issues, and major administrative decisions. In order to meet these issues directly, it is necessary to confront and negotiate so that the issues can be resolved in a limited time. No one person always functions within one leadership style, but one style usually predominates. Weiss states that the best way to involve others in a cause demands that the leader develop a style in which she is comfortable and then act that way most of the time (14). By doing this, followers generally have more positive feelings and are thus more willing to be led by this leader. Leaders who are flexible, however, are able to move from style to style as the situation necessitates. For example, the team leader who generally functions as a democratic leader finds she must become autocratic in an emergency situation. The effective leadership approach used by a head nurse in attempting to foster leadership development within her staff under particular circumstances may be the laissez-faire style, in order to stimulate thinking and bring forth spontaneous reactions. This contingency or situation leadership pattern is the most effective, but it takes an understanding of leadership styles and experience with them to make use of such an approach.

Characteristics associated with the autocratic leader are based on the person's concern about the job. Frequently the leader is insecure and tries to compensate for that insecurity by putting forth a firm approach as the sole source of authority, the final decision maker. This type of person would prefer to work alone, but her leadership position forces her to delegate functions. As a result, all details for each task are specific, with little time or patience for questions or discussion because she is the sole authority in the area. This type of person tends to see the staff members as lazy, needing close observation and frequent criticism. This is a reflection of McGregor's Theory X (see Chap. 8). Although there appears to be high productivity with the autocratic leader, there is a high incidence of staff turnover and perhaps a large number of grievances, both of which take time from the day-to-day activities of a busy unit. Staff members can lack motivation, and creativity is not usually facilitated when this autocratic style predominates.

If one attempts to seek acceptance of a new idea by the autocratic-style leader, the best approach is to lay the groundwork subtly, providing factual data and background information, so that the leader will feel secure in giving an affirmative response. If it can be arranged so that the leader perceives this new idea as hers, the problem is solved; she will direct that it be carried out.

Further along the leadership style continuum is the bureaucratic leader, similar to the autocratic leader in that she is insecure and finds security in following the policy manual accurately. This type of leader wields her power by fixed rules and is deficient in initiative and flexibility. There can be no variation or exceptions from what is stated in print, the interpretation of which is usually very narrow and leaves no question in the reader's mind. As long as the rules are followed, there are no problems. If new ideas are to be accepted by this kind of person, the best approach is to show how these new ideas remain within the framework of the stated policies. If the idea requires a broader interpretation of policy, the use of informal channels of communication to plant the ideas with people who have the respect of the bureaucratic leader may be helpful. These people may have a greater impact in assisting with a broader interpretation and implementation of policy.

At another point on the continuum between the bureaucratic and the democratic leaders is the mollifying autocrat, who is concerned about too much independence within the staff but is also concerned about the staff as people. This person usually communicates well with the staff, listening to what they have to say, asking their ideas. Once they have had an opportunity to speak and feel they were heard, this leader goes ahead and does what she had planned prior to discussion with the staff. The mollifying autocrat frequently has great skill in changing the mind of those in disagreement in a manipulatory way. The following is an illustration of how this approach works. Two faculty members who expressed their concern about a double standard of punishment meted out to two students for infraction of the same rule, were asked by the nursing administrator of the hospital to discuss this problem. Having had discussions with the administrator on previous occasions, the faculty members spent some time planning how they would present their concerns. At the outset they were given an opportunity to present their case, the administrator listening attentively. The presentation was followed by some comfortable discussion about the problem during which the faculty felt they had gotten across their point. An hour after the conference began, the two faculty members started to leave the office thinking they had succeeded in changing the administrator's mind, only to realize that gradually the administrator had changed what they had said to agree with her own philosophy. The administrator had used effectively the technique of manipulation of meanings of words. The faculty found themselves agreeing with her statements yet were opposed to them philosophically.

The democratic leader is a secure person who sees the staff as self-reliant. She works with the group to set objectives and allow the staff to plan ways to meet them. She is usually an open person who welcomes the introduction of new ideas. Such an atmosphere nurtures a highly motivated, creative staff with high job satisfaction. The one drawback of this style of leadership is that the decision-making process takes longer than with the other styles of leadership. However, depending on the situation, the positive factors far outweigh any negative outcome. In emergency situations, a democratic leader may have to take an autocratic approach temporarily, but this behavior usually will be positively received by staff due to the urgency of the situation and the normally consistent style of the leader.

The last leadership style is laissez-faire. In this instance, the leader has no set goals or policy. The nursing staff is free to do what it wants. The effectiveness of the staff will depend upon the people within the group. If there is no strong person, the group is essentially leaderless and the staff flounders. In many instances, an informal leader takes over and the unit runs smoothly when that person is there, as the staff looks to her for guidance. When raising new ideas, it is important for the informal leader to validate findings and have strong rationale because this liassez-faire leader will not interfere or introduce change unless there is a problem — and even then she becomes upset if she is pressed to accept the responsibility and must be accountable for the actions of her staff.

According to Weiss (15, p. 31), leadership can be very situational. What is occurring at the moment can involve more than the leader's usual behavior. Therefore, the leader should consider four major factors when determining her style: the time available, how critically committed to the issue others are; whether the issue includes role expansion for others, and where the expertise to resolve the issue lies.

The experiences of nurses at one management workshop serve as an example of the effectiveness of the three major styles of leadership. The nurses were divided into three groups. A leader was appointed in each group, and all leaders were given the same instructions for the group: they were to draw a picture of a house, in ten minutes. The directions for each leader varied, one being autocratic, one democratic, and one laissez-faire. The outcome of the groups with autocratic and democratic leadership usually were predictable. Members of the group with autocratic leadership finished the drawing quickly, often within five minutes. Their drawing lacked imagination and usually included only the house. When asked how they felt about the experience, the participants said they felt frustrated, angry. Some sat back and would not participate unless it was demanded of them. They said they did not feel a part of the experience and were dissatisfied with the product, that it was all work, no fun.

Frequently the group members with democratic leadership did not quite finish the drawing. They took time to decide what they wanted to do and how to divide the work. While working, they had pleasant conversation about the task, with suggestions being offered to one another. The drawing was almost always detailed, including curtains, door knobs, and landscaping. One group produced an underwater habitat. They all had a good feeling about their *product*. People from this group often continued conversing with their new colleagues after the exercise.

The outcome of the laissez-faire group was never predictable. In one instance, each person in the group drew her own house. In a second group, a leader emerged when she could no longer stand the nonproductivity of the "leaderless" group. She became an autocratic leader so that the group could meet the deadline. When the group discussed their reaction, they said they were angry and frustrated with the appointed leader because she was of no assistance. At first they were grateful that a leader emerged, but they did not like her style.

In summary, each professional finds herself in a leadership role, at some level, each day. The style of nursing leadership and its effectiveness are inherent in the leader's demonstration of behavior related to each component of the nursing leadership process. To be the most effective leader, she must know her own preferred style and be able to adjust this style so that it is most effective for a given situation. She can be an autocratic, democratic, or laissez-faire leader if she understands the advantages and difficulties inherent in each style, as well as the possible variations. In addition, she must recognize that situations determine the need for one style over the other. Her predominant style and the emphasis on the people with whom she works will help her to motivate these people by her enthusiasm and a feeling that she works with them and will support them. As a result, the staff will feel comfortable with her as a pace setter, trusting her judgment as well as her actions, and responding to her effectiveness as a leader with creativity, productivity, and a general feeling of self-worth.

REFERENCES

1. Yura H, Ozimek D, Walsh MB: *Nursing Leadership Theory and Process.* New York, Appleton-Century-Crofts, 1976, p. 121.
2. Merton RK: Leadership, in Stone S, et al (eds), *Management for Nurses.* St Louis, CV Mosby, 1976, p. 98.
3. Stevens W: *Management and Leadership in Nursing,* New York, McGraw-Hill Book Co, 1978, p. 124.
4. Gill W: Key concepts in management nursing. *Supervisor Nurse* 2:21, September 1971.
5. Tannenbaum R, et al: *Leadership and Organization.* New York, McGraw-Hill Book Co, 1961.
6. *Webster's New World Dictionary,* 2nd college ed. New York, World Publishing Co, 1970, p. 862.
7. Letterer VA: *Organization: Structure and Behavior.* New York, John Wiley & Sons Inc, 1963, p. 141.
8. Beach DS: *Personnel: The Management of People at Work.* New York, Macmillan Inc, 1965, p. 425.
9. Cartwright D, Lippitt R: Group dynamics and the individual, in Hill and Egan (eds): *Readings in Organizational Theory: A Behavioral Approach.* Boston, Allyn & Bacon Inc, 1966, p. 251.
10. Peterson GG: Power: a perspective for the nurse administration. *J Nurs Adm* 9:7, July 1979.
11. Alexander E: *Nursing Administration in the Hospital Health Care System.* St Louis, The CV Mosby Co, 1972, p. 244.
12. Donovan HM: *Nursing Service Administration.* St Louis, The CV Mosby Co, 1975, pp. 8–9.

13. Leininger M: The leadership crisis in nursing, *Nurs Adm* 4:29, March-April 1974.
14. Weiss AJ: Surviving and succeeding in the "political" organization: becoming a leader. *Supervisory Management,* p. 30, August 1978.

BIBLIOGRAPHY

Periodicals

Adkins R: Responsibility and authority must match in nursing management. *Hospitals* 53:69–71, February 1979.

Colton MR: Nursing's leadership vacuum. *Supervisor Nurse* 7:29, October 1976.

Courtade Sr Simone: The role of the head nurse: power and practice. *Supervisor Nurse* 9:16–23, December 1978.

Erickson EH: Are nurses needed for administration or management in hospitals? *J Nurs Adm* 4:20, July-August 1974.

Fiedlaer FE: The trouble with leadership training is that it doesn't train leaders. *Psychology Today,* p. 23, February 1973.

Gill W: Key concepts in management in nursing. *Supervisor Nurse* 2:20–21, September 1971.

Hershey P, et al: A situational approach to supervision's leadership theory and the supervising nurse. *Supervisor Nurse* 7:17, May 1976.

Hershey P, et al: A look at your supervising style. *Supervisor Nurse* 2:64, January 1971.

Hooper SA: Becoming an administrator — overnight! *Nurs Outlook* 23:752, December 1975.

Kolba TM Sr: The human equation in supervision. *Supervisor Nurse* 2:64, January 1971.

Kron T: How to become a better leader. *Nursing '76,* p. 67, October 1976.

Leininger M: The leadership crisis in nursing: a critical problem and challenge. *J Nurs Adm* 4:28, March-April 1974.

Levenstein A: The art and science of supervision: role ambiguity in nursing. *Supervisor Nurse* 7:16, June 1976.

McClelland DC, Burnham DH: Good guys make bum bosses. *Psychology Today,* p. 69, December 1975.

McNally JM: Gentleness, an attribute for administrators. *Supervisor Nurse* 7:65, October 1976.

Marriner A: Theories of leadership. *Nurs Leadership* 1:13–17, December 1978.

Pike D: Management theory: its application to the job. *Supervisory Management* 23:26–30, December 1978.

Schweiger J: Dealing with apathy in nursing. *Supervisor Nurse* 7:42, July 1976.

Singleton JP: Managing versus management by results. *Supervisory Management* 24:31–37, May 1979.

Thompson K, Pitts RE: The great balancing act. *Supervisory Management,* pp. 22–29, May 1979.

Weiss AJ: Surviving and succeeding in the "political" organization: becoming a leader. *Supervisory Management,* pp. 27–35, August 1978.

Zaleznik A: Managers and leaders: are they different? *Harvard Bus Rev,* pp. 67–78, May-June 1978.

Books

Alexander E, *Nursing Administration in the Hospital Health Care System.* St Louis, The CV Mosby Co, 1978.

Beyers M, Phillips C: *Nursing Management for Patient Care,* ed 2. Boston, Little Brown & Co, 1979.

Brooton D, Hayman L, Naylor M: *Leadership for Change: A Guide for the Frustrated Nurse.* Philadelphia, JB Lippincott Co, 1978.

Ganong J, Ganong W: *Nursing Management, Concepts, Functions, Techniques and Skills.* Germantown, Md, Aspen Systems Corp, 1976.

Stevens W: *Management and Leadership in Nursing.* New York, McGraw-Hill Book Co, 1978.

Tannenbaum R, Weschler I, Massarik F: *Leadership and Organization.* New York, McGraw-Hill Book Co, 1961, p. 263.

Yura H, Ozimek D, Walsh MB: *Nursing Leadership Theory and Process.* New York, Appleton-Century-Crofts, 1976.

5. Inter- and Intradepartmental Communication

"Tune In or Tune Out"

Joyce L. Schweiger, R.N., M.S.

BEHAVIORAL OBJECTIVES

After reviewing this chapter, the reader will be able to

- identify specific communication techniques and their application to personnel situations within a bureaucratic structure
- recognize the need for close interdepartmental relationships
- describe the importance of the exchange of ideas among various departments within the health care agency
- use the expertise of personnel from other departments in planning innovative methods of providing care

Communication can unite people. It is a means of expression that will either close or widen a gap, depending upon the manner in which it is given and received. Generally, communication is defined as giving and receiving information, signals, or messages by either talking, gesturing, or writing. Pluckhan (1) further clarifies the meaning by describing it as a process that is complex, dynamic, transactional, and highly unpredictable.

Communication has always been a basic component of nursing. Nurses are dependent upon messages sent to and received from peers, superiors, clients, and all members of the health care team. The question is, "How well do we communicate?" Do we take the time to analyze all the variables that communication encompasses? Do we unthinkingly say words and send messages and then wonder why the recipient is unreceptive and confused? Our ability for self-expression does not prevent us from unknowingly erring and causing a communication lag, that, if not rectified, leads to a gap. The gap is a tune-out mechanism that can be attributed to a lack of understanding of the three areas crucial to communication:

1. words and language
2. use of words
3. elimination of barriers to effective communication

WORDS AND LANGUAGE

Language is one way to formulate ideas and communicate them. Language sets the tone for good communication in the hospital and outside environment. Errors in either words or language occur because of the lack of a complete data base. The recipient is not receiving a complete message printout from the sender. Confusion is the result. Four of the basic concerns in language and words are

1. how we use words
2. how we listen to words
3. how we react to words
4. how we send words

How We Use Words

An error in word choice or an omission of words can alter the meaning and context of a communication. Predetermined conclusions without investigation can add to the complexity of a comparatively trivial situation. For example: A nurse sees a man wearing only a patient gown walking toward the maternity department. She does not approach the gentleman to question him, but calls security to report the incident. Security responds promptly. The security officer asks the nurse where the man has gone. The officer is directed to the men's bathroom, where he encounters the gown-clad intruder and asks: "Hey, Bud, what are you doing up here?" The gentleman answers: "What do you mean, what am I doing up here? I'm here to see my wife. She had a baby two hours ago." The security officer asks him why he is walking through the halls wearing a patient gown. The new father replies that he was directed by a nurse to "Go into that room, put on a gown, and then you may see your wife." The new parent followed instructions, but the nurse who gave them omitted important words related to the dress code. The gown was to be worn over his clothing. The nurse who saw the father later jumped to conclusions and called the security officer, who assumed he would encounter an unstable person. If the first nurse had given clear directions and had taken time to be certain that the new and excited father understood, an awkward and embarrassing situation would have been avoided.

Accustomed to giving directions to staff familiar with hospital policies and procedures, nurses sometimes fail to recognize that to the uninitiated — that is, a patient or visitor — the hospital is a complex and unfamiliar setting. Nurses fall victim to what Pluckhan (1, p. 115) describes as dysfunctional communication — that is, a failure to get the response from a message that the sender expected.

How We Listen to Words

Listening is not an innate ability but is attained over time and with experience. In some instances, the ability is never achieved.

Does the listener receive what the speaker is sending? Listening and hearing are two different activities. Listening may be more than a matter of the person's being quiet and attentive when information is presented. There are variables to consider.

One variable is a bias in listening — that is, what we hear is not always what is said. This bias occurs when the listener has preconceived ideas and opinions about the topic being discussed. A second variable relates to the manner in which the material is presented. The presentation format offers the listener the opportunity to read between the lines, even though a hidden message may not be there. The third variable is the objectivity of the listener. One rarely listens with total objectivity. As the message is received by the listener, it becomes intertwined with the recipient's ideas, feelings, and attitudes, whether they are positive or negative.

Hopefully, the listener is able to separate feelings, ideas, and attitudes from content and weigh them accordingly. The ultimate success of the sending-receiving process is dependent upon how the information is finally interpreted by the listener. Because the listener is habitually conditioned to think beyond the spoken word, she will probably decide to accept or to reject the message either before or after the delivery of the message.

One example of the process in action is the relay of information through established communication channels in a nursing department. The director of nursing receives a written communication from the hospital administrator. The director calls her administrative team together and verbally transmits the information she has received. They, in turn, are instructed to "pass it on" down the line via the usual channels—for example, head nurse to staff nurse, and so forth. How much content is lost with this verbal transfer of communication will be based on how well listening processes function. The only evaluation of the staff's listening abilities is through the feedback that eventually reaches the administration. Feedback appears in verbal return, attitude, and performance. Problems often can be avoided if the manner in which the original communication is given is approached in three steps: in writing, by verbal reinforcement, and by accurate interpretation. In each instance, time is allowed for the recipients to digest the information, question it, and respond to it. Clarification at the first level results in less confusion and/or misunderstanding as the information passes through the channels to all involved. In some instances, tape recorders can be used to ensure accuracy of meaning before information is released. By playing back the tape, the initiator is able to react to what he has said. Understand what is heard and interpreting it correctly promote the internal cohesiveness of the organization.

How We React to Words

Society today is engulfed in commercial advertising used by the news media to provoke attention. Titles of books, films, or plays do not necessarily reveal the content and, at times, leave one confused. We are victimized frequently by catchy phrases. The health care field is no exception. For example, a physician tells his patient, "You have malignant hypertension," and proceeds to discuss the problem. The patient didn't hear the word *hypertension;* he heard only the word *malignant,* and to him this means cancer. In this situation, the words caused a volatile response, one that could have been avoided if the thought process had been used before the word process. The physician could have told that patient, "You have a high blood pressure that is causing some damage to your blood vessels." Everyone tends to react spontaneously to the unknown and unclear. Medical or technical terms should be explained before or when used. Words mean different things to different people (see Fig. 5-1).

The skill of producing or receiving an appropriate reaction to words used is developed by getting to know the audience. To do this, learn to

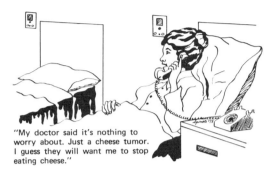

"My doctor said it's nothing to worry about. Just a cheese tumor. I guess they will want me to stop eating cheese."

Figure 5-1. "Cheese tumor."

1. Recognize the person's level of comprehension.
2. Be aware of the level of anxiety that the information you provide may evoke.
3. Know the person's cultural background, since it may strongly affect his response.
4. Be sensitive to body language. For example, if the person is quiet and apparently receptive in manner, it may seem that he is handling the transfer of information with relative ease. However, his body language — rigid posture, clenched fists — may communicate a very different message.

The transfer of information between people can be an involved process. The receiver's perception of what he hears and what its meaning is frequently differs from that of the presenter. The manner in which words are chosen can make the difference between a successful or unsuccessful nurse-to-patient, patient-to-physician, or peer-to-peer interaction. The overall effect can be a lasting one. In the instance of the patient-to-nurse interaction, it is crucial to remember that, in the agency setting, the person who has either voluntarily or by necessity been placed in the nurse's hands presents a different aspect of himself than when he is on familiar, safe, home territory. This reaction to words is not new since we all have, at one time or another, experienced it in either our professional or personal lives and responded accordingly. The key in reacting to words is the word choice of the speaker.

How We Send Words

It is equally important to send the complete meaning of a message. For example, a nurse tells her patient, "I'll bring your pain medication right away." She intended to do exactly what she said, but she forgot that the unexpected occurs frequently in the clinical setting and the timing of events is uncertain. It would be better to say: "I will get back to you with your pain medication as soon as I can. If I do not return within ten minutes, please call."

The importance of sending a verbal message accurately is significant not only because of the immediate effect it has upon the recipient—in this situation, a person in pain—but because it reaches further and deeper than a superficial interaction. It affects the trusting relationship between the nurse and the patient. This is important, not only in the nurse-patient relationship, but in all aspects of daily living. Opinions formed by recipients when they receive unclear, direct verbal messages frequently remain unaltered. The sender finds that, in all future interactions, either competence must be proved or integrity defended. Neither is a suitable solution.

If we take the time to consider how we use words, how we listen to words, how we react to words, and how we send words, we can effectively strengthen and improve interpersonal relationships.

USE OF WORDS

Words don't stand alone. They need support. The supports are

1. clarification of the word meaning in context
2. distinction of the word in presentation
3. individuality of people

Clarification of the Word

An elderly woman was taken to an outpatient eye clinic at a large inner city hospital. Her niece accompanied her. While they were waiting to be seen by the physician, the medical clerk gave the patient a sheet of paper and asked her to "Please fill this form out. We need it for your record." The 82-year-old woman obliged and, with her niece's assistance, proceeded to fill out the patient history sheet. Suddenly, she stopped, rather firmly placed the pen on the desk, and said, "I will not fill this paper out." When asked why, she replied: "It says here what are my complaints? I have never complained about anything in my life, and I am not here because I have a complaint. I am here to see a doctor because I have trouble seeing." Eventually, after some prodding and explaining by both the niece and the clerk, the form was completed.

Had the meaning of the word *complaint* been explained to the patient before handing her the history sheet, the embarrassing event would not have occurred. We establish a code of communication in our personal and professional lives. If we do not make those we wish to communicate with aware of what our particular code is, uncertainty of meaning, misinterpretation, confusion, and, as in the above example, anger can result. Meaning, again, is not solely in the word, whether it is verbal or written, but in how the word is used in context. The word cannot stand alone.

Distinction of the Word in Presentation

This support refers to directive and informative statements. For example, the head nurse attends a meeting where a new policy that she is to put into effect as soon as she can is introduced. She returns to her floor to share the information with the staff. There are two approaches that she can use.

In the first approach, she would say to the staff: "Starting Monday you will be doing problem-oriented charting on every patient. If you haven't seen the film on the process, you will have to work it in. It will probably have to be done over your lunch hours. Everyone will be doing problem-oriented charting, and the nursing supervisors will be checking."

Using the second approach, she would say: "Today in our head-nurse meeting we talked over the possibility of introducing problem-oriented charting. We have been discussing the advisability of introducing this procedure for a long time, and we feel that now is the time to initiate it. We realize that everyone on the staff has not seen the descriptive film on the tapes or read all the available information. Therefore, each unit will have to work this out to fit their schedule. It may have to be done on an individual basis. In order to initiate this procedure, I have set an initial target date, which is *four weeks from Monday*. This, I feel, will allow everyone adequate time to iron out details."

The *directive approach* used by the nurse in the first example is inappropriate. It should be used in a situation that calls for quick thinking and immediate action, such as an emergency. The *informative presentation* used in the second example is the more democratic way to introduce or change policy. Informative presentation should be the primary method of verbal interaction in both individual and group communications.

Individuality of People

It is a common tendency to generalize in conversation. As a professional, one should be particularly aware of this tendency and try to avoid it. Never say, "*All* gall bladder patients are going to be nauseated"; or "You shouldn't be having trouble; the patient down the hall had surgery two days ago, and he is up and walking in the halls"; or "It will never work; it never has in the past."

Each person and each situation is unique. Individuality must be recognized and identified. Labeling has no place in effective communication, and generalization falls into this category.

ELIMINATING BARRIERS TO EFFECTIVE COMMUNICATION

Eliminating barriers to effective communication is the final crucial area to consider in developing effective communication skills. This area encompasses

1. clarifying unclear self-expression
2. being aware of peripheral barriers, noise, and interruptions
3. identifying lack of interest or preoccupation with topic
4. being aware of overthinking or wordiness process

Clarifying Unclear Expression

Clear expression concerns everyone within the health care system. This concern includes administration, physicians, nurses, all allied health care workers, and particularly the recipient of the care—the patient. Intelligent verbal and written communications are the basic components of clarity of expression. The following directive received from administration illustrates the havoc that can result when written communication is neither clear nor complete: "Subject: Fire Drill. A fire drill will be held Wednesday, October 10 at 9:00 A.M. The staff on 3-North will report to the northwest area, and the staff on 3-West will report to the southwest area." This directive may result in confusion among the nurses because few or none may be certain which area is north, south, east, or west. A diagram accompanying the memo would have made the communication more effective.

Being Aware of Peripheral Barriers—Noise and Interruptions

Noise is at the top of the list of criticisms from patients who complete questionnaires about their hospitalization. "It was too noisy in the hospital, I went home to rest" is heard too often.

Telephones and intercoms are recognizable barriers to a quiet hospital but are, of course, not readily eliminated. Loud communications and conversations among professionals in the corridors also draw frequent complaints. This noise can be minimized if consultation rooms are used to advantage.

Interruptions are not conducive to establishing good communication with the patient. For example, there are peripheral interruptions, such as a volunteer offering magazines, a ward assistant filling water pitchers, and a ward secretary delivering mail during a nurse's visit with a patient. These apparently insignificant annoyances can interfere with the development of a nurse-patient relationship. The nurse who thinks and plans her schedule and routine can alleviate this interruption barrier. For example, she is well tuned into hospital routine. She knows that at "coffee break time" the number of ancillary personnel interacting with the patient will be minimal. Therefore, she may choose that time to deliver specific information to the patient.

Identifying Lack of Interest or Preoccupation with the Topic

This practice is common among the professional staff, as well as between staff and patients. The nurse whose basic concern is speed rather than effective performance may not be interested in and may resent answering questions of a new staff member who may not be familiar with the hospital's routine procedures. The answers this nurse gives may be superficial and lacking in detail. Inadequate exchange of information at this level could cause confusion with the new nurse and, more importantly, with the patient under her care. A broad example would be a policy stipulating that all patients will have diagnostic procedures explained to them unless otherwise specified by the physician. This procedure may not be a common practice in all hospitals, and may not have been routine procedure to the new nurse. If this detailed information was overlooked by the preoccupied nurse, the result could have been an unnerving reaction by the uninformed patient; and because the new nurse did not explain a diagnostic procedure, the omission also may have resulted in an unwarranted reprimand to the uninformed nurse.

Being Aware of Overthinking or the Wordiness Process

Specific messages or directions may, many times, be lost in too many words. Directions to staff or communications to patients very often relay unpleasant information. The nurse may become so engrossed in what to say and how to say it that the message is lost. For example, a patient was told that chemotherapy would be started. The physician informed the nurse that chemotherapy was scheduled for his patient but that the patient was not told when it would begin. The nurse was not told the details of the physician's conversation with the patient. She did not know the patient's reaction to the information and, as a result, she spent all her time contemplating how the patient would accept this turn of events. Her concern increased and, by the time she delivered the message, the information was muddled, redundant, and meaningless to the patient. She said: "I guess the doctor spoke to you about your treatments. They'll be starting very soon." Her concern for the patient was so overwhelming that she overlooked the basic requirement of a message—simplicity. A few words can relay a message or answer a question. Weil (2) quotes Edwin Newman's example of verbiage in *A Civil Tongue,* which is not hospital-oriented but exemplifies this point clearly. President Ford, when asked by a reporter whether he had the brains to be president, replied: "My feeling of security, my feeling of certainty grows every day. I feel very secure in the capability that I have to do the job." He could have said, "Yes, I can do it," or even "Yes."

The three basic areas in communication—words and language, use of words, and elimination of barriers to effective communication—that were applied to a professional setting are also applicable in daily life.

Some other aspects to consider are the intricacies of inter-intra departmental communication within the bureaucracy of the hospital setting. There are four major concerns:

1. communication patterns
2. relationship between managers at all levels
3. vehicles for transmitting information in a hospital bureaucracy
4. long-term and short-term goals of the health care agency

The communication pattern among managers is dependent on their primary relationships. Primary relationships refer to face-to-face interactions. The first primary group in the health care agency consists of the administrator and the directors of the agency's services. Primary relations involve tensions, as well as positive responses, but they cannot survive in an atmosphere of antagonism. The primary relation fosters a sense of belonging together and a sharing of a common interest. Verbal sharing at this level will ensure effective performance because subordinate groups will follow the example.

The second primary group in the nursing department is the supervisors and head nurses. The relationship this group projects should be based on harmony, and will reflect the attitude and leadership style of the director of nursing. Harmony can only be established in a setting where mutual respect, flexibility, understanding, and pride exist; where there is concern for each person. Without harmony we invite mistrust, and the best-established communication system will falter.

Attitude sets the tone among managers and between managers and staff. If a manager is an isolate and withholds communications, she will be displaying an attitude that may be interpreted as noncaring, and this attitude can have far-reaching consequences. The staff and level associates will interpret noncaring as negativism, which may eventually affect their attitude and performance.

The leadership style of the director cannot be overlooked. The interest and concern she displays in her interpersonal actions directly affect the attitude and performance of all nursing personnel. If she establishes an open-door policy as a means of communication with her staff, there will be a free flow of information, both positive and negative, that will stimulate ideas, invite creativity, and encourage critical thinking. This may seem to be an impossible policy to uphold, but a leader who has chosen the administrative nursing team with care and good judgment is able to delegate responsibility. She can then rely upon feedback, which will allow her to activate her policy rather than have it appear only as hearsay.

The open-door policy is one vehicle for facilitating communication flow within the bureaucratic setting. Another highly effective method of transmitting information and enhancing communication skills is through seminars, workshops, lectures, and the use of available current literature. Establishment of an active and knowledgeable staff development team can determine which vehicle would be most effective in the specific agency.

A final factor in bureaucratic communications, not to be overlooked, is the involvement of all personnel in all departments at all levels in the planning and implementation of short- and long-term goals. This personnel involvement and participation will enhance the quality of these goals and expedite their attainment.

From the basic concepts to the intricacies of communication in the hospital organizational setting, the effective sharing of information among peers, supervisors, and physicians is a real accomplishment. If communication is out of tune within the organization, the sound will be heard as a note of discord throughout management and staff. This is why it is important to think, rethink, and then communicate.

REFERENCES

1. Pluckhan ML: *Human Communication: The Matrix of Nursing.* New York, McGraw-Hill Book Co, 1978, pp. 9–11.
2. Newman ER, quoted by Weil AW, in Clean up your language. *Consulting Engineering* 50:16, May 1978.

BIBLIOGRAPHY

Periodicals

Beard JM: What is your attitude saying? *Association of Operating Room Nurses* 24: 782–788, October 1976.

Cuthbert BL: Switch off, tune in, turn on. *Am J Nursing* 69:1206–1277, 1969.

Fry WF, Lauer J: The planning team: why include nursing membership. *J Nurs Adm* 11:70, 1972.

Goodwin L, Taylor N: Doing away with the doctor-nurse game. *Supervisor Nurse* 8:25, June 1977.

Griffith K: Interpersonal trust in the helping professions. *Am J Nurs* 69:1491–1492, 1969.

Levenstein A: The art and science of supervision: mind your language. *Supervisor Nurse* 7:50, December 1976.

Marriner A: Organizational process and bureaucratic structure. *Supervisor Nurse* 8:54, July 1977.

McConnell EA: What's the difference? *Supervisor Nurse* 7:20, November 1976.

McWilliams RM: The balance of caring. *Association of Operating Room Nurses* 24:314–323, August 1976.

Nash AI: Conflict relations between nursing supervisor, practical nurses, attendants. *J Nurs Adm* 7:9, July-August 1977.

Shubin S: Communicating (or, make that non communicating) with doctors. *Nursing '79* 9:89, February 1979.

Smith C: Identifying blocks to communication in health care settings and a workshop plan. *Continuing Ed in Nursing* 8:26, 1977.

Stein LI: The doctor-nurse game. *Am J Nurs* 68, January 1968.

Wicker IB Jr: Cultural barriers to employee communications in the hospital. *Supervisor Nurse* 2:32, July 1971.

Books

Blake RR, Moriton JS: *Guideposts for Effective Salesmanship.* New York, McGraw-Hill Book Co, 1978.

Donovan HM: *Nursing Service Administration, Managing the Enterprise.* St Louis, The CV Mosby Co, 1975, pp. 33–37, 48–49.

Newman E: *Strictly Speaking.* New York, Warner Books, 1974.

Pluckhan ML: *Human Communications: The Matrix of Nursing.* New York, McGraw-Hill Book Co, 1978.

Robinson L: *Psychological Aspects of the Care of Hospitalized Patients,* ed 3. Philadelphia, FA Davis Co, 1976.

Rosenberg SL: *Self-Analysis of Your Organization.* New York, AMACOM, 1974, pp. 133–166.

Stone S, et al: *Management for Nurses: A Multidisciplinary Approach.* St Louis, The CV Mosby Co, 1976, pp. 49–57.

6. Problem Solving

"An Active Exercise"

Joyce L. Schweiger, R.N., M.S.

There is no more miserable human being than one in
whom nothing is habitual but indecision.

William James (1)

BEHAVIORAL OBJECTIVES

After reviewing this chapter, the reader will be able to

- utilize the principles of problem solving
- compare and contrast the methods of problem solving
- identify variables that affect the problem-solving process
- identify the obstacles to problem solving
- solve problems by using the seven-step method

From infancy to death the two constants we face in our lives are that of decision making and problem solving. Ironically, they are the issues that we at times and for varied reasons attempt to circumvent, avoid, overlook, or refuse to recognize as existing. Nursing devotes a large percentage of time to problem solving at all levels and in various degrees.

Problem solving appears in the literature under many names and the literature contains many sources that offer different problem-solving methods and approaches. Allen Morgenson refers to the problem-solving process as work simplification, "organized use of common sense to find easier, better ways of doing work" (2). Donovan equates problem solving with the nursing process that Carlson describes as "the sum of the activities jointly performed by the patient and the nurse" (3) — that is, assessment of the patient, problem identification, development of a plan of care, and evaluation of the care plan's effectiveness. Kron (4) refers to problem solving as systematic thinking, sometimes called the scientific method of thinking.

Before we can apply any one or all of the approaches to problem solving, we must be certain of one thing. Do we have a problem? If we do, how do we recognize it? Is it an intuitive reaction? Does it stem from the way someone looks at us? Is it sudden realization that comes to us while we're planning our activities of daily living?

McCool and Brown (5) give two essential clues to problem awareness: (1) environmental monitoring (EM) and (2) delineation of issue.

Environmental monitoring involves recognizing a deviation from the normal course of events. It depends on the development of sensitivity to people, places, and things. For example, you are talking with a person, not on a face-to-face basis but by telephone; when you call, the person's voice carries an unusual inflection. You immediately identify a deviation from the normal. You have been made aware of something that is not quite as it should be; you have carefully monitored your environment without too much effort and found a change.

The second clue, delineation of issue, involves the *awareness* that a problem exists, and implies that the person is capable of more than just recognizing signs and symptoms, that he is able to comprehend the issue in its entirety and do something about it (5, p. 102). This type of awareness makes it necessary to put the problem into words to determine the how, what, when, where, why, and who of the situation.

Several tools are available to assist the decision maker in objectively evaluating whether a problem exists. One tool familiar to many nurses is the nursing process, a variation of the classic scientific method. Health professionals must be able to adapt the method to any situation that arises and to pursue those steps that will help solve the immediate problem (6).

THE PROBLEM-SOLVING PROCESS

The problem-solving process in itself comprises seven steps. The person using the process will dictate the degree of effort and attention to be paid to each step depending upon her experience, position, and the scope of the problem.

The seven steps to problem solving are

1. identification of the problem

2. analysis of the problem objectively
3. exploration of the alternative solutions
4. selection of the most fitting alternative
5. consideration of consequences
6. implementation of the solution (decision)
7. evaluation of the solution

Identification of the Problem

Does the problem really exist? How do you know? What is wrong? A problem generally arises when a need is not met or fulfilled. This need could be personal or professional. Baily and Claus (7) define a problem as a discrepancy that exists between what actually is and what should or could be.

Does the incident that represents a problem suggest a deviation from the goals and objectives that have been predetermined? Is there enough data collected and presented to justify that a problem exists? Do the data collection and examination of the data reflect a deviation? As the data are presented or reviewed, the recipient must listen, think, and rethink carefully to determine the validation that has accompanied the data. Remember that to oversimplify or repress a problem can lead to greater and more complex problems that could lead to deleterious outcomes for the person or persons involved.

Another approach to determine the existence of a problem is through the development of a model, a diagram of the incident that has occurred. On the diagram, specify what has happened, when did it happen, how did it happen, who was involved, where did it happen, and has it ever happened before? If so, how frequently? Are you dealing with a transient issue or one that has recurred time after time but has never been verbalized? In the incident diagram, place this information in the appropriate category so that the collected data will appear in a more objective format for evaluation. The cliche "seeing is believing," in this instance, does have some merit.

Analysis of the Problem

If you are satisfied with the information you have received from the problem identification, you are ready to approach the second step — analysis of the problem. This should be done as objectively as possible. Objectivity is difficult to maintain, particularly if you have already formulated an opinion in regard to the problem. Brown expresses it quite capably when he says: "Looking for facts is like walking in a circle in the forest. One never gets a chance to see how the trees look from the other side" (8).

Be certain the presented facts are relevant to the issues. We cannot do very much without the support of facts, but Brown (8, p. 212) suggests that they can lead us into difficulties if we are not aware of their weaknesses. Facts can: (1) influence us too much, if we stand too close; (2) be negative in character; (3) be closely identified with destruction rather than construction; (4) be past-oriented; (5) show things after the fact; (6) be one-sided — show what happened, not what could happen; (7) be whimsical — facts don't change (we do, and we change facts to meet our needs); (8) be presented in a seductive manner and lead to anxiety; (9) be taken out of context; and (10) be hard, impersonal, unfeeling.

Careful assessment of facts, with these points in mind, will provide the decision maker (problem solver) with insight into determining what is relevant for use in forming alternative solutions to the problem.

Exploration of Alternative Solutions

In exploring alternative solutions to the problem, *do not* belittle the way the problem has been handled previously if it is a recurring one. Some problems are long-standing before they reach you, and attempts already have been made to resolve them. The methods used in the past do not warrant an open critique on your part. Such criticism may result in lack of support for your solution if you say the method used was outmoded, a poor idea, or showed a lack of good judgment.

Approach the search for solutions in a methodical way. You can, for example, determine if there is a policy that may serve as a guideline for action in the situation. If such a policy exists, review it. A discussion of the policy with appropriate personnel may result in a change in or an addition to the existing policy. This will improve its applicability to future situations of the same nature.

If there is no existing policy to work with, draw upon the existing expertise on the staff to find a solution. Involve the staff members at the grassroots level in addition to those in administrative roles. The same principle applies to problem solving as to management by objectives. Solutions, like goals, are developed from bottom up as well as from top down. If you do invite participation, do not ignore the suggestions from the group. If the problem has had a direct effect on the staff, their solution may tend to be less objective, but this does not necessarily negate the solution they propose in its entirety. It only may need some refinement.

Another method to employ in exploring solutions to the problem is to rely upon past experiences in similar situations. This does not always supply an answer, but it could aid in the thinking process. Do not neglect to investigate other sources for ideas. Review the literature, attend relevant seminars, hold brain-storming sessions or use the inductive-deductive reasoning process. While you are investigating one or more of these methods, a solution may be discovered that is new and innovative. If it is workable and effective, this will be most rewarding to the problem solver.

In the search for possible solutions, one usually finds more than one alternative, particularly when several people are involved and more than one method is employed. The decision is to select the one solution most applicable to your situation.

Selection of the Most Desirable Alternative

After investigating all the parameters to determine a solution that seems to be the most satisfactory, choose one and test it. Before submitting it as the probable solution, do more than make an armchair review. Invite critique from outsiders. A consultation with an outside professional who has been faced with similar problems would provide an unbiased objective opinion, and perhaps it would make you recognize variables within the solution that you had not considered. You can also put the tentative solution to a written test. Just as you diagrammed the problem, diagram the solution. Write the problem down with all the alternatives that have been suggested, and from this determine if the alternative that has been selected seems the most fitting in your situation and setting.

Take a positive attitude toward your solution; you will need it when it is put into effect.

The majority of creative solutions to problems do not come from mind grinding, but will usually surface at a point and time when least expected. If you are convinced that you have the best solution, consider the consequences.

Consideration of the Consequences

In considering the consequences that may result because of the solution you have chosen, attempt to look at the solution with two thoughts in mind. First, there are no perfect solutions; and, second, not every problem is solvable, and you may have to compromise.

The consequences, either positive or negative, that result because of your solution will depend upon the nature of the original problem. You may have to concern yourself with patient safety, staff acceptance, cost, possible failure of the solution. You must return to the beginning problem process and ask yourself: Will the solution decided upon accomplish the objective? Will the solution be effective and efficient? How soon can it be implemented? After you have answered these questions, implement the solution.

Implementation of Solution (Decision)

Successful implementation of the solution (decision) will again depend upon to what extent coworkers or staff have been considered and involved, along with the material components. When the solution is implemented, do not ignore voices that express concern about the decision. Listen to the concerns, and hear the fears, for apprehension is a major block to progress and could stalemate it. Since you are the implementor, take a few precautions.

- Introduce the solution to the primary group involved. This can be done through workshops, seminars, consultant speakers, or informal discussions and feedback critiques.
- Be certain that all who will be affected by the solution are informed, both verbally and in writing, *before* the solution is implemented.
- Set a time that is agreeable to the majority involved with the problem for implementing the solution.
- If the problem is one that has affected many clinical areas, select one area agreed upon by the majority as a trial area to implement the change. This gives you an opportunity to even out rough spots, and allow for any extraneous variables that you may have overlooked. Then after a trial period, involve the entire department if the problem was one that encompassed all areas.
- Finally, wait for feedback. It will come via many routes, and will be both positive and negative. This is what you want — an input from those who are directly involved.

Evaluation of the Solution

After the solution has been implemented for a reasonable length of time in all areas involved, evaluate its effectiveness. Do not forget that the problem existed. Do not write it off as solved. If you do, it will resurface. The length of time allowed for implementation of the solution will depend upon how serious and how far-reaching the effects of the initial problem were, as well as how much time or how many people were involved. Three months is usually an acceptable length of time to determine the success or failure of the solution, with an interim report six weeks after implementation.

OBSTACLES TO PROBLEM SOLVING

Problem solving is not easy. An awareness of obstacles on the part of the decision maker can ease the transition from step to step in the problem-solving process.

The goal of obstacle awareness is to motivate the individual faced with problems continually to be aware of possible extraneous variables, no matter how large or small the problem appears to be.

There is little doubt that in the list compiled below you will find familiar obstacles to problem solving. Most of them can obstruct solutions to personal as well as professional problems. They are

1. stress
2. oversimplification
3. personality
4. inadequate data base
5. time
6. emotions
7. information source
8. placating

Stress

Selye defines *stress* as "the nonspecific response of the body to any demand made upon it" (9). A nonspecific response refers to a demand for readjustment. In other words, the agents we are exposed to under stress require or demand an increase in body response to perform adaptive functions and reestablish normalcy. Many times we are presented with a problem to solve and a decision to make; but at the time of presentation of the issue, we are under stress. It may be personal or professional stress that has taken its toll in spite of the fact that we believe we have a reserve to fall back upon and that, after a little rest, we can pick up where we left off. It may seem that stress has not noticeably left its mark, but it has. Longevity of life can be affected by the presence of stress and how the individual handles it.

For example: You have just left the monthly department-head meeting and the controller discussed the budget, always a touchy subject for nursing service. He asked that everyone begin the task of determining needs so that budget plans can be made and priorities set. After a morning of this, your thoughts bound ahead. You know what you need and are aware of what the staff wants. You recognize that a great deal of planning must be done prior to any workable budget agreement. This realization immediately causes you stress. In this frame of mind, you return to your office. You are approached by a staff nurse who is off duty but has to see you regarding a personal problem that is infringing upon her performance. Right now you have no time to discuss her problem or share your opinions with her, and yet you profess to have an open-door policy to employees. This situation produces a second stress in a short period of time. You become agitated, preoccupied, and ambivalent about your feelings. The person before you is also demonstrating stress, and you know that you should not compound the situation. What should you do?

First, put your last meeting aside for the moment. Second, take care of this nurse's immediate needs. She needs a listener: listen and empathize. Then arrange a more appropriate time (and there always is one to be found) to meet her needs so that you can help her to solve her problem.

Oversimplification

Oversimplification frequently occurs when the individual involved is faced with solving a problem, and lacks either time, patience, or both. When a real problem presents itself, the person, if he is busy and preoccupied with other matters, may belittle the situation. He may dismiss it with a wave of the hand and a simple "That's not too difficult, just do thus and so." If the person lacks time and patience to investigate all parameters of the problem, he may hasten a solution by making a quick decision himself or cause those who have presented evidence of the existing problem to make an an immediate decision based on suggestions he has made without any consideration or thought of the outcomes. The primary danger with oversimplification is that the problem is not solved. It is merely shuffled, placed farther down the ladder of concerns until some issue stimulates it again and it has to be reconsidered. Hopefully, the second time around the decision maker will not employ the same technique. However, that depends upon the decision maker.

Personality

The personalities of the people involved easily influence or affect the problem-solving process. Unfortunately, we are not always as impartial as we like to think we are in situations. We pride ourselves as professionals, believing that we are tolerant and open-minded at all times. This is a fallacy. Problems that are brought to us are not always presented to us by a personality type that we look upon favorably. You can recall situations when someone told you equipment was needed and care could not be given in an effective way, so that there seemed no alternative but to purchase new or additional equipment. This is not an unfamiliar request and, in many cases, is a legitimate request. Is your response legitimate? Is your decision ever affected by the personality of the person who has brought the problem to you? Has she been a professional threat to you? Is she usually negative in her approach to others? Is this the person who always has a better plan, an easier way of doing things when new policies or procedures are introduced? Answer these questions fairly and honestly before you make a decision. See the problem and all of its ramifications in a nonjudgmental way.

Lack of Data

Accepting problem information from just one or two sources may make the problem appear small and inconsequential and readily resolved. However, failing to get all the facts and rendering a decision without them may compound the issue and cause a small ripple to develop into a tidal wave. The important thing to remember is that the accumulation of a firm data base will allow you to reject or eliminate unnecessary or noncontributing information. Collecting data takes time, but in the end it will save time. A decision made with all the relevant data at hand is usually a permanent one.

Time

We never seem to have enough time. We are always marking it, working against it, trying to buy more. However, in the problem-solving process, time must be given its just due. Speed is only appropriate in an emergency situation. Quick settlement is inappropriate in long-range planning and can result in a trial and error method, so that the decision becomes vulnerable.

Take as much time as you need; do not be rushed by those who are attempting to project their wishes or thinking on you. Do set a limit on your time. Have your solution ready when you say it will be ready. Do not try to buy time by procrastinating or pushing the problem aside. Many managers have a habit of falling into this pattern so that problems either are never resolved or become so compounded that all perspective is lost, and immeasurable and irrevocable damage results. Time is only an obstacle if you make it work as one.

Emotions

Emotions can influence what one thinks he saw or heard. Emotions can interrupt the problem-solving process in two ways: first, if the person presenting the problem is emotionally involved; and, second, if the recipient of the information or problem is affected by the emotional overtones. Frequently, our immediate response is tinged with emotion, but let it be a salient response if at all possible. Emotional reactions, outbursts, and tirades may cloud the issue. At times it is advisable to move away from the situation. Reflect—then ask: what occurred? Why did it occur?

Emotions may cause us to override reason and choose solutions that have no firm foundation.

Information Source

Source of information overlaps the obstacle of personality influences—with one exception—what or who was the original source of the problem data? Was it from several sources, formal (head: nurse meeting, nurses' staff meeting) or informal (coffee breaks or the grapevine)? Knowing the exact source of information can lead you to determine if you really have a problem to be solved or if it is one of those many circles that form when we skip stones across the water.

Placating

Do not appease, mollify, or pacify anyone while using the problem-solving process. This clouds the issue, dampens the facts, drowns the alternatives, and leaves you with a lukewarm solution. It is ineffective.

If you try to avoid these obstacles to problem solving while you are systematically using the process described earlier in the chapter, your efforts to reach workable solutions are likely to meet with success.

REFERENCES

1. James W, in Peter LJ: *The Peter Prescription.* New York, William Morrow & Co Inc, 1972, p. 156.
2. Ferguson SA, Womer CB: Work simplification in the worker's job. *Modern Hospital* 87: 61, 1956.
3. Donovan H: *Nursing Administration — Managing the Enterprise.* St Louis, The CV Mosby Co, 1975, pp. 22–23.
4. Kron T: *The Management of Patient Care,* ed 4. Philadelphia, WB Saunders Co, 1976, pp. 51–52.
5. McCool B, Brown M: *The Management Response: Conceptual, Technical and Human Skills of Health Administration.* Philadelphia, WB Saunders Co, 1977, pp. 101–104.
6. Sorensen, K, Luckmann J: *Basic Nursing: A Psycho-Physiologic Approach.* Philadelphia, WB Saunders Co, 1979, p. 256.
7. Baily JT, Claus KE: *Decision Making in Nursing.* St Louis, The CV Mosby Co, 1975, p. 21.
8. Brown RE: *Judgment in Administration.* New York, McGraw-Hill Book Co, 1966, p. 211.
9. Selye H: *Stress Without Distress.* Philadelphia, JB Lippincott Co, 1974, pp. 27–28.

BIBLIOGRAPHY

Periodicals

Daniel WW, et al: An introduction to decision analysis. *J Nurs Adm* 8:20, May 1978.
Erickson EH, Bergmeyer V: Simulated decision making experience via case analysis. *J Nurs Adm* 9:10, May 1979.

Fredette S: Problem solving with a difficult patient. *Am J Nurs* 77:622, April 1977.

La Monica E, Finch FE: Managerial decision making. *J Nurs Adm* 8:20, May-June 1977.

Marriner A: The decision making process. *Supervisor Nurse* 8:58, February 1977.

Stevens BJ: The use of consultants in nursing service. *J Nurs Adm* 7:7, August 1978.

Taylor AG: Decision making in nursing: an analytical approach. *J Nurs Adm* 8:22, November 1978.

Books

Alexander EL: *Nursing Administration in the Hospital Health Care System,* ed 2. St Louis, The CV Mosby Co, 1978.

Bailey JT, Claus KE: *Decision Making in Nursing.* St Louis, The CV Mosby Co, 1975.

Beyers M, Phillips C: *Nursing Management for Patient Care,* ed 2. Boston, Little Brown & Co, 1979.

Brown RE: *Judgment in Administration.* New York, McGraw-Hill Book Co, 1966.

Donovan HM: *Nursing Service Administration — Managing the Enterprise.* St Louis, The CV Mosby Co, 1975.

Kron T: *The Management of Patient Care,* ed 4. Philadelphia, WB Saunders Co, 1976.

McCool B, Brown M: *The Management Response: Conceptual, Technical and Human Skills of Health Administration.* Philadelphia, WB Saunders Co, 1977.

Shanks MD, Kennedy DA: *The Theory and Practice of Nursing Service Administration,* ed 2. New York, McGraw-Hill Book Co, 1970.

Stone S, et al: *Management of Nurses: A Multidisciplinary Approach.* St Louis, The CV Mosby Co, 1976.

7. Change Without Disruption

"The Need to Plan Ahead"

Mary Ann Miller, R.N., M.S.N.

BEHAVIORAL OBJECTIVES

After reviewing this chapter, the reader will be able to

- identify those influences that promote change in nursing
- identify those influences that cause resistance to change
- identify how strengths can be maximized and forces of resistance minimized in situations of planned change
- devise a plan for change in nursing practice using principles of the change process

Today hardly a meeting or conference takes place without some mention of the challenge of change. People cope with this loss of permanence in many different ways. Some deny its existence, some resist it with every effort, struggling to maintain the status quo. Some people manage to cope with the change they initiate but resist change initiated by others. Some people see in change a challenge to be overcome, and they actually welcome its presence.

Almost everyone experiences some degree of discomfort when faced with any change. This discomfort produces energy, and how this energy is channeled can be crucial to the success of the change process. This is especially true in nursing, where members of the profession are faced with changing philosophies of care as well as changing technologies. Influences outside the profession that force these alterations include the changing role of women in society, a more sophisticated public, increased involvement in medical affairs by government and community groups, advances in medical technology, and the emergence of new paraprofessional roles. Within the profession, there is sometimes conflict surrounding the expanded role of the professional nurse, her licensure, or her entry level into practice. There are new means of evaluating care that is given and of evaluating the care giver as well. There has been a change in nursing's focus, from a negative self-image perpetrated by years of subordination demanded by those in authority positions to a positive self-image encouraged by the current movements in consumerism and women's rights. In reaching this positive self-image, nurses have become more aware of not only their clinical strengths and weaknesses but also of their personal energy and willingness to risk making changes and to take full responsibility for the consequences. Today nurse power is becoming a reality (1).

THE CONCEPT OF CHANGE

Change may be defined as any significant alteration in the status quo. It occurs when there is an imbalance in the forces working toward maintaining the current situation and the forces working toward disrupting it. Changes often are described as major or minor, although what one person considers a minor change may be seen as a major change by someone else. Effects of change can rarely be isolated, since they will have an impact on the immediate as well as the adjacent environments. What changes have you had to cope with in the past year, month, week? A change from team nursing to primary nursing? Writing nursing histories for patients? Doing problem-oriented charting? Participating in peer evaluations? Working with a new head nurse? Moving to a new unit? Trying a new technique that is supposed to result in better patient care? How did you react when you were faced with some of these changes? How did others react? Were the changes planned? Did the changes just happen?

METHODS OF CHANGE

Many times change is recognized only in retrospect as people have responded to forces such as personalities, aging, finances, or legislation without realizing that change is occurring. Change of this nature may be referred to as "organizational or institutional drift" (2). Everyone has been a passive participant in this type of change.

There is also the traditional approach to change described by Bennis (3). This approach is based on the assumption that ideas change the world and, therefore, the emphasis is placed on direct teaching, on propagandizing, on advertising.

Planned change utilizes an approach that is distinct from the traditional approach and is the ideal method. It involves a problem-solving process with specifically identified elements. There is deliberate collaborative action directed toward a cause or goal with an identified change agent (or agents) to advance the cause. Distinct channels of action in which to employ specific strategies are chosen by the change agent. The change agent may function as a catalyst, getting the change started and helping to provide a group atmosphere in which the change can occur. The change agent may be a solution giver, sharing ideas about what needs to be done and how it can be accomplished. The change agent may actually assist the group move through the change process (4). Many times it is helpful if the change agent is an outsider, independent of the current situation and free from emotional ties to the personalities involved or to the status quo. On the other hand, the change agent can be a member of the organization—for example, the staff nurse or the nurse manager.

FIRST PHASE OF THE CHANGE PROCESS

In order for change to begin, the change agent (or agents) must define the stress or need that exists. If there is no need, then there is no reason to make a change. Change should be planned to reduce the stress or to satisfy the existing need. For example, the nursing staff may not be satisfied about the care that patients are receiving. They see nursing care as fragmented, with no one person ultimately responsible for the care of the patients. The stress is dissatisfaction, and changes are planned in an attempt to reduce that stress. Those changes may range from minor modifications in the existing traditional team approach to nursing care to the adoption of a system of primary nursing. If, however, the team approach is working effectively and both staff and patients are pleased with the care being given, a change to primary nursing just because it is the latest trend would be extremely disruptive. No one would be satisfied, and a great deal of energy would be channeled toward defeating the change.

Once the need for change is felt, the nurse-manager (or change agent at any level) can stimulate an awareness of this need among members of the group and let them know that better conditions are a possibility. This sets the stage for the first of Lewin's (5) three phases of change — "unfreezing" — during which forces are mobilized in the direction of producing the change and helping, collaborative relationships are formed.

SECOND PHASE OF THE CHANGE PROCESS

Defining the Problem

In the next of Lewin's phases — "movement" — the problem is identified, alternative solutions are explored, goals and objectives are set, and a plan to reach the goals is implemented. First, as the problem is defined, the discrepancy between what is and what should or could be becomes clear. Claus and Bailey (6) recommend answering eight questions in order to provide definite parameters for the problem: what is happening? (what is not happening?), where is it happening? (where is it not happening?), when is it happening? (when is it not happening?), what is the extent of the happening? what is the nature of the happening?

Assessing the Environment

Once the problem is defined, the change agent assesses the total environment for existing resources supportive of change and resistive to change. If she is wise, she makes special note of the existing power/authority structure and includes people from that group in the planning or decision-making process. She also approaches people from various interest groups who will be touched by the effects of the change, and she solicits their input (6, p. 36). She approaches her own colleagues, seeking their ideas and cooperation in the planning process. She keeps all interested parties aware of the facts through the use of a well-planned communication system. This is perhaps the most important element to be considered if the change process is to have a chance of being successful. Clear communication channels ensure that there are no surprises for anyone and that each person has an opportunity to state his opinion. This is vital if forces of resistance are to be minimized as much as possible (7).

Forces of resistance to any planned change are always present and have recognized causes (8,9). Resistance may increase if the nurse-manager or change agent fails to be specific in describing a change, fails to show why a change is necessary, or fails to allow those affected by the change to have input into planning for it. The change agent who meets resistance is likely to have used only personal appeal to gain acceptance of the change or to have disregarded a work group's habit patterns. She has probably failed to keep employees informed about the change or to allay their fears about possible failure if they must master new skills. She may have failed to deal with their anxiety over job security, or she may unknowingly have created excessive work pressure during a change if it was not planned far enough in advance or if too many changes were planned for the same time.

As Stevens (10) points out, the change agent can avoid such problems by trying to provide answers to the following questions that those affected by the change are likely to have: Will the change cause my position to be different? Will it increase or decrease my power? Will it increase or decrease my status? Will the content of my job be different? Will new activities be added? Will I have more or less freedom to determine how I will do my job? Will job inconveniences be relieved? Will my financial status be improved? What benefits does the proposed change offer to me? What benefits do I have now that might be taken away?

One of the most frequent causes of employees' resistance is uncertainty about how they will be affected personally by the change. This is especially obvious when a major change occurs, such as the appointment of a new superior, whether it is a new hospital executive director for the director of the nursing department or a new head nurse for the staff on a particular unit. The more directly a person sees himself affected by the change, the greater is his uncertainty about his future.

Another very frequent concern is that the change will be inconvenient. It is viewed as creating more work or requiring more energy or greater concentration. An example of this occurred with the adoption of the nursing history as a tool to gather patient data. When this idea was first introduced, many nurse-administrators met with resistance from their staff. Staff members saw this method as extremely time-consuming and creating more work for already overworked personnel. This type of resistance might have been averted if staff members had been made aware of the ultimate benefits to be derived from the use of nursing histories.

Objectors to change frequently point to resulting increased costs in time or money. Anyone seeking any change that involves expenditure of funds should be able to defend the added expense in terms of increased benefits, especially if there are economic benefits over a period.

The economics of time itself proved to be an important factor in one institution where the medication administration system was changed to reduce medication errors. Instead of finding medication records on the patients' charts, physicians had to consult with the medication nurse, who had the medication records. Because the physicians found this too time-consuming, they resisted the change and through increased pressure caused the old medication procedure to be reinstituted. The real obstacle here was a lack of communication with the physicians before the change was instituted. If they, as members of the health team, had been made aware of the benefits expected from the change (a reduction in medication errors) and had been included in the planning process, their resistance probably would not have been as vigorous.

A number of general approaches are helpful for the change agent to use in reducing resistance to change. First, she must be sure that the change is necessary. She will find that resistance to the proposed change is decreased if she can stimulate some interest in it among the people who are to be affected by the change and can give thoughtful consideration to their comments about the proposal. She should be able to demonstrate that the change has administrative support; that it will offer tangible benefits, such as reducing the work load rather than increasing it; that it takes employees' existing values and ideas into account; that it does not threaten employees' autonomy and security. Resistance will be less if the people involved have participated in the planning process and recognize the importance of the proposed change; if they have had the freedom to air their objections in an accepting atmosphere; if they have experienced confidence and trust in their relations with one another; if the project is kept open to revision and no irreversible decisions are made (8, pp. 22–24). If the change agent is aware of the danger of these pitfalls, she can avoid most of them with a little effort and achieve a large benefit.

Choosing a Strategy

The change agent uses certain tools in working with others to achieve change. These range from persuasion to influence to force (10, p. 59). Persuasion has two components that may be used singularly or together—reason and emotion. Reason involves the intellectual approach, providing all possible data that support the change in the hope that the people involved will see the change as necessary. When change is initiated at the staff level, persuasion through reason is essential. It proves that the change agent has done her homework and knows her facts. Her presentation should include a rationale for the change, both positive and negative aspects of the change, and alternative methods of reaching the goal.

Reason alone is not effective in bringing about acceptance of change if those involved in the change have a strong emotional investment in the status quo. The issue of smoking is a good example. When the No Smoking campaign began, the primary thrust was to persuade the public not to smoke by giving all the facts about what smoking would do to a person's life span and what diseases it might cause. The ineffectiveness of the rational approach can be seen by the increase in smoking, particularly among young girls. The campaign has shifted now to persuasion through emotion. Because popularity among peers is so important to teenagers, smoking is being depicted as dirty, unsophisticated, and unacceptable. Within the nursing profession, persuasion, through a combination of reason and emotion, can be very effective in bringing about change. A sound scientific rationale should always be the basis for any proposed change, but the power exerted by emotion should not be neglected.

Influence is another strategy for implementing change. Influence is a stronger force than persuasion since it does not require the argument of a cause. Influence exists because of some power associated with people, either formally by virtue of the office they hold or informally by virtue of the esteem in which they are held. (These are not mutually exclusive.) Informal power is one of the keys to the success of the change process. If those who will be affected by the change respect the person who is initiating the change, the process is likely to occur more smoothly and with less resistance.

If it is the position that commands respect rather than the person in that position, the change is likely to be more disruptive. Although change may occur, it may not be the change intended. For example, the director of the nursing department in a large metropolitan hospital was never seen on the units and was not well respected generally among the nursing staff. With no advance warning, she called the staff of an acute care unit together and told them that, within four weeks, the unit would admit only patients needing ambulatory care. Since the unit would be staffed almost totally by nonprofessional nurses, the professional nurses would be reassigned to other larger units throughout the hospital where registered nurses were in demand. The nurses knew that the shift rotation schedules on these other units were less desirable than the schedules they were on currently. With even a cursory analysis of this situation, it becomes clear that many of the requirements for successful change were ignored. No one was informed of the change before the announcement, opinions were not solicited, participation in planning was not invited, the change clearly was not to the benefit of the registered nurse staff, and no sound rationale for the change was offered to the group. The proposed change did occur; the focus of the unit did change as the director ordered. However, as a result of the way the change was handled, five of the seven RNs who were to be reassigned submitted their letters of resignation and obtained employment elsewhere. If the goal of the change was to obtain more RNs for other units, it missed its mark.

Selecting a Solution

Once the change agent has analyzed the human and material environment into which the defined change is going to be introduced, the implementation process begins. The best solution to the problem is chosen from several alternative approaches based on past experience and knowledge, the advice and recommendations of experts, and the collective expertise of all those involved in planning the change (6, pp. 36–37). This best alternative is the one that is most likely to achieve the expected outcomes, which are stated in clear behavioral terms. It is these objectives against which the success of the change will be measured. Claus and Bailey (6, p. 59) detail specific steps to be taken during the implementation of the change. Plans should be carefully written, tasks should be clearly defined, and the person who is to carry them out should be clearly designated. Reporting procedures and communication channels should be determined so that progress can be shared. Change agents should follow up on communications so that the danger of misinterpretation or misunderstanding among those concerned can be reduced. A specific time limit should be set for the project and, within that time frame, specific reporting dates should be chosen so that progress can be periodically and systematically evaluated.

Positive considerations at the point of beginning implementation include the possibility of doing a pilot study of the change on a unit that is conducive to a trial run and over a period that is long enough to give the change an opportunity to succeed. The staff on this unit should be aware of the influence the trial will have on the final decision regarding widespread implementation of the change. That influence should be considerable if maximum support by the staff is desired. If the staff feel that their opinions will carry weight in the final decision-making process, they will be more willing to offer suggestions for solving any problems that arise during the trial run. In addition, if major alterations have to be made, fewer people will have to cope with the modifications and run the risk of developing negative attitudes toward the change. After modifications in the plan are made as indicated, the change is instituted on a wider scale, evaluated, modified as necessary, and finally accepted.

THIRD PHASE OF THE CHANGE PROCESS

Lewin's (5) third phase in the change process is that of "refreezing" — the change is integrated into present behavior and is no longer questioned or criticized. This may occur sooner than expected if the timing of the steps of the change process has been appropriate, if persuasion and influence have been used effectively, and if the environment generally has been supportive of creativity and innovation (see Fig. 7-1).

This chapter has dealt primarily with methods a nurse-manager or change agent might use to bring about change. It is also worthwhile to consider what our responsibilities are when we are the participants in the change process rather than the initiators of it. Approach the change with an open mind and a willingness to try something new and different. Seek as much information about the change as possible. Ask questions. Take time to evaluate both the positive and the negative aspects of the change. Try to offer only constructive criticism and make certain that your feedback is communicated to the appropriate people through appropriate channels. Remember that, when change is inevitable, efforts to maintain the status quo waste far more energy than efforts to achieve a smooth transition. By holding disruption to a minimum, we can use that energy to provide quality nursing care.

REFERENCES

1. Bowman R, Culpepper R: Power: rx for change. *Am J Nurs* 74:1053–1056, June 1974.
2. Reinkemeyer A: Nursing's need: commitment to an ideology of change. *Nurs Forum* 9:344, May-June 1970.
3. Bennis W: New role for behavioral science. *Adm Sci Q* 15:130–134, September 1963.
4. Gibson C: The concept of change. *Maine Nurse* 4:15, July 1973.

Change Agent(s)	Change Participants

Unfreezing
Identify the need for change.
Stimulate awareness of the problem.

Be open to new ideas and willing to participate.

Movement
Define the problem and anticipated outcomes of the change. Change only what is. Collect facts to justify the change.

Seek information.
Contribute ideas and feelings about how you will be affected.

Assess the environment. Identify forces of support. Include them in planning. Include power/authority figures. Include persons from interest groups affected by the change. Include colleagues. Identify forces of resistance. Work to minimize them.

Establish clear channels of communication. Keep all interested and involved parties informed of progress.

Seek answers to questions using appropriate channels.

Examine alternative solutions to problem.

Contribute ideas using appropriate channels.

Choose best solution from all alternatives.

Choose strategy for implementation of change.

Write the plan, including measurable objectives. Who will do what and when? When and how will each step be evaluated?

Institute trial run.

Participate in change. Offer constructive criticism.

Give positive reinforcement to participants.

Make modifications based on evaluation.

Institute on a larger scale. Give positive reinforcement to participants. Modify as necessary based on ongoing evaluation.

Refreezing
Accept change in daily practice.

Accept change in daily practice.

Figure 7-1. Steps in the process of change.

5. Lewin K: Group decision and social change, in Maccoby E, Newcomb T, Hartley E (eds): *Readings in Social Psychology*. New York, Holt, Rinehart & Winston, 1958, pp. 210–211.
6. Claus K, Bailey J: Facilitating change: a problem-solving/decision-making tool. *Nurs Leadership* 2:35, June 1979.
7. Douglass L, Bevis E: *Nursing Leadership in Action*. St Louis, The CV Mosby Co, 1974, pp. 170–173.
8. Lippitt G: Managing change: six ways to turn resistance into acceptance. *Supervisory Management* 11:21–24, January 1966.
9. Watson G: Resistance to change. *Am Behavioral Scientist* 14:745–765, May-June 1971.
10. Stevens BJ: *The Nurse as Executive*. Wakefield, Mass. Contemporary Publishing Inc, 1975, p. 58.

BIBLIOGRAPHY

Periodicals

Ashley J: About power in nursing. *Nurs Outlook* 21:637–641, October 1973.
Bolman F: Problems of change and changing problems. *J Higher Ed* 41:589–598, November 1970.
Bunning R: Changing employees' attitudes. *Supervisor Nurse* 7:54, May 1976.
Cleland V: Implementation of change in health care systems. *J Nursing Adm* 2:64–69, November-December 1972.
Day H: Change can be planned and effected. *Supervisor Nurse* 5:47–49, March 1974.
Fischman F: Change strategies and their application to family planning programs. *Am J Nurs* 73:1771–1774, October 1973.
Ganong W, Ganong J: Motivation, Maslow, and me. *Supervisor Nurse* 4:25–32, July 1973.
Guerin Q: A functional approach to attitude change. *Management Rev* 59:33–37, August 1970.
Heineken J, Mussbaumer B: Survival for nurses initiating change. *Supervisor Nurse* 7:20, October 1976.
Leary P: The change agent. *J Rehab* 38:30–33, January-February 1972.
Leininger M: Conflict and conflict resolution. *Am J Nurs* 75:292–296, February 1975.
Levenstein A: Effective change requires change agent. *Hospitals* 50:71–74, December 1976.
Lysaught J: No carrots, no sticks, motivation in nursing. *J Nurs Adm* 2:43, September-October 1972.
Marriner A: Planned change as a leadership strategy. *Nurs Leadership* 2:11–14, June 1979.

Peterson G: Power: a perspective for the nurse administrator. *J Nurs Adm* 9:7–10, July 1979.

Pierce S, Thompson D: Changing practice: by choice rather than chance. *J Nurs Adm* 6:34–39, February 1976.

Rodgers J: Theoretical considerations involved in the process of change. *Nurs Forum* 12:160–174, March-April 1973.

Ruano B: This I believe . . . about nurses and innovating change. *Nurs Outlook* 19:416–419, June 1971.

Schaefer M: Managing complexity. *J Nurs Adm* 5:13–16, November-December 1975.

Schlotfeldt R: Planning for progress. *Nurs Outlook* 21:766–769, December 1973.

Schlotfeldt R, MacPhail J: An experiment in nursing: introducing planned change. *Am J Nurs* 69:1247–1251, June 1969.

Shirley R: An interactive approach to the problem of organizational change. *Human Resource Management* 14:11–19, Summer 1975.

Smith D: Change: how shall we respond to it? *Nurs Forum* 9:391–399, July-August 1970.

Smoyak S: The confrontation process. *Am J Nurs* 74:1632–1635, September 1974.

Soltis F: A systemic approach to managing change. *Management Rev* 59:2–11, September 1970.

Stevens BJ: Management of continuity and change in nursing. *J Nurs Adm* 7:15–17, April 1977.

Books

Arndt C, Huckabay L: *Nursing Administration: Theory for Practice with a Systems Approach.* St Louis, The CV Mosby Co, 1975.

Bennis W, Benne K, Chin R: *The Planning of Change,* ed 2. New York, Holt Rinehart & Winston, 1969.

Brooten D, Hayman L, Naylor N: *Leadership for Change: A Guide for the Frustrated Nurse.* Philadelphia, JB Lippincott Co, 1978.

Clark C, Shea C: *Management in Nursing.* New York, McGraw-Hill Book Co, 1979.

Lewin K: *Field Theory in Social Science.* New York, Harper & Row, 1951.

Stevens BJ: *First-Line Patient Care Management.* Wakefield, Mass, Contemporary Publishing Inc, 1976.

Stevens W: *Management and Leadership in Nursing.* New York, McGraw-Hill Book Co, 1978.

8. Staff Motivation

"A Rolling Stone . . .?"

Mary Lou Hamilton, R.N., M.S.

BEHAVIORAL OBJECTIVES

After reviewing this chaper, the reader will be able to

- identify selected theories of motivation
- identify varying needs in people that require satisfaction in order to develop job productivity
- define the term *motivation*
- list two types of motivational style
- discuss thirteen ways a nurse-manager can motivate a nursing staff to accept responsibility for improved patient care

Theorists as well as observers of human behavior have implied that people are motivated to grow and produce their best when they have a part in the planning and decision-making activities involved in their growth or production process. People are motivated to perform any activity when they can have freedom of choice to set the goals they desire to complete the activity. When working in conditions in which there are incentives, people are interested in completing organizational goals by using creative, imaginative, and carefully developed techniques in cooperation with other employees. There are times, however, when certain factors interfere with the completion of an organizational goal, causing frustration or blocking, and employees seem to be unmotivated to perform.

THEORIES OF MOTIVATION

Motivation is a quality that is present in varying degrees in different people. It is determined by individual needs and desires, the physical conditions of the job, and the social conditions of the job. Satisfying a person does not necessarily motivate her to improve her performance and contribute to greater productivity. The relationships among need satisfaction, morale, job performance, and productivity are very complex and influence the degree of motivation in the person. People seem to be motivated by what they are seeking much more than by what they already have.

According to Alexander, theorists Maslow, Herzberg, and others provide the framework for looking at the monetary, security, power, competence, status, and achievement motives of all people in a modern organization (1). Their theories can be readily applied to any nursing situation.

THE MONISTIC THEORY

The monistic theory is based on principles of scientific management. Frederick Taylor, a mechanical engineer who experimented in management techniques, described this theory. He discovered that some quality was needed if an energetic man with high productivity learned that he earned no more than a lazy worker who did as little as possible; as a result, the energetic man lost interest in producing his optimum (2). Taylor decided that to prevent this loss, incentive was needed. The incentive could be in the form of payment for piecework. A larger paycheck would increase one's self-esteem and provide a type of status to the worker. What Taylor had not counted on was that the constant competition and pressure placed on the worker to produce so much caused tensions that often led to undesirable behaviors. He concluded that the amount of motivation provided by money is questionable.

THE HIERARCHY OF NEEDS THEORY

A. H. Maslow outlined his basic motivational model in 1943 and said that a person's motivational needs could be arranged as a hierarchy. When a person's needs are met at a certain level, they no longer serve to motivate. The next level need must then be activated in order to motivate the person (3).

Figure 8-1 illustrates the leveling of needs from the most basic to the highest and most fulfilled and illustrates the steplike procession to self-fulfillment that each person may decide to undertake (4). According to Maslow, a person moving up the hierarchy may reverse direction and move downward if his lower-level needs are in jeopardy and cannot be met. The closer to self-fulfillment the person gets, the more difficult the process becomes. Complete self-fulfillment is rarely attained.

A summary of the five basic needs identified by Maslow follows.

1. *Physiological integrity (survival needs)*. Survival needs are needs for food, water, oxygen, elimination, rest, exercise, sex, shelter, and protection from the elements. These needs are independent of each other but must be met continuously for the person to remain fulfilled. Marriner suggests that the more a society becomes affluent, the less do physiological needs serve as motivators (5). Hospitalized patients, at times, do have these needs thwarted and, as a result, demonstrate behaviors that demand attention by a nursing staff.

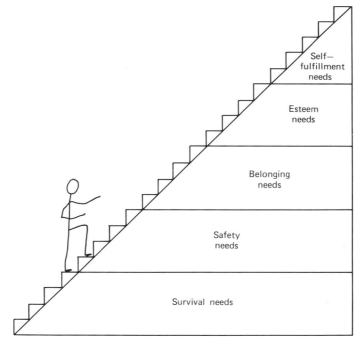

Figure 8-1.   The hierarchy of needs.

2. *Safety needs.* Safety needs include a need for a stable environment in which threats of danger and deprivation are not present. Safety needs are activated by such qualities of administration as arbitrary management actions, employee discrimination, unpredictable policy, and favoritism. In the health care setting, a nurse may feel threatened when she does not feel qualified to care for a complex patient. A patient may feel threatened when placed in an involuntary dependency relationship or when faced with a frightening diagnostic test, such as a breast biopsy.

Safety needs do not usually become motivators unless the person is seriously threatened or endangered (4, p. 147). Then, needs for safety may completely dominate the person, causing severe anxiety, fear, and behavioral reactions that are difficult to control.

3. *Belonging (love) needs.* Belonging needs include feelings of belonging, acceptance by one's peers, recognition as an accepted member in a group, being an important part of an activity, giving and receiving friendship, and affectionate relations with others (5).

People, because of their social nature, usually want friendship and companionship. When working toward a mutual goal or objective, workers who belong to small integrated work groups have higher morale than those who work alone. Teamwork is often necessary for good morale. Thwarting of social needs by management or other groups can stimulate resistance and antagonism, as these thwarting actions appear as personal threats.

Studies such as those conducted by Hawthorne in 1927 point out that workers often resist being in competition with their peers and consciously or unconsciously tend to band together to resist anything from management that may appear as a threat to the individual (4, p. 147). For example, meeting group norms may become very important to a person as experienced by the head nurse on a medical surgical unit. Her nurse's aides are a compatible group in the coffee-break room, and they seem to spend a great deal of time there. In fact, they would rather take extended coffee breaks than perform routine nursing functions. If, however, one aide is willing to complete her nursing assignment ahead of time and without the usual coffee breaks, she is seen to be rejected by her aide-peers and classified as a "do-gooder," with comments to the effect that she is "too self-righteous" for the rest of the group.

4. *Esteem needs.* Achievement, competence, knowledge, independence, status, recognition, prestige, appreciation, reputation, and respect all contribute to self-esteem and confidence. It is helpful if management tries to meet these needs by using pay raises, titles, and constructive evaluations when deserved. Unlike the lower-level needs,

esteem needs are not easily satisfied. These needs appear greater in high achievers, professionals, and highly skilled workers. They might appear more as motivators among head nurses and supervisors in a health care institution.

5. *Self-fulfillment or actualization needs.* Most writers of motivational theory agree that a person never achieves all of which he is capable. Such feelings as accomplishment, responsibility, importance, challenge, advancement, and new experiences, including opportunities for growth, help contribute to self-fulfillment. Beyers and Phillips list qualities that Maslow describes the self-actualized person as having (4, p. 148):

- superior perception of reality
- increased acceptance of self, others, and nature
- increased spontaneity
- increased problem-solving ability
- increased detachment and desire for privacy
- increased autonomy and resistance to enculturation
- greater freshness of appreciation and richness of emotional reaction
- higher frequency of peak experiences
- increased identification with the human species
- changed interpersonal relations
- more democratic character structure
- greatly increased creativeness
- certain changes in the value system

For a discussion of these qualities, the reader is referred to Maslow's original work (6). An understanding of Maslow's needs theory helps us see that needs overlap but that the lowest-level needs never really disappear. Each higher need level emerges before the lower ones are completely satisfied. Most people tend to have more satisfaction at the lower need level. An understanding of need theory is helpful to nurse-managers in building goals and objectives in their personal work and in planning and implementing leadership skills to motivate other employees.

HERZBERG'S THEORY OF MOTIVATION

In 1950, Frederick Herzberg conducted studies on work motivation and developed the two-factor theory, which is closely related to Maslow's need hierarchy (7). Herzberg reduced Maslow's five levels to two and divided his theory into *hygienic factors* (*dissatisfiers*) and *motivator factors* (*satisfiers*). *Hygienic* factors include preventive and environmental aspects such as supervision, policy, salary, and working conditions. Herzberg suggested that these factors do not necessarily lead to satisfaction and become motivators, but they must be present to prevent dissatisfaction. *Motivator* factors such as achievement, recognition, work responsibility, and advancement really do motivate people on the job.

The healthy worker wants a balance between hygienic and motivator factors. She wants a pleasant environment yet, at the same time, needs to feel she can accomplish and be creative. In 1959, Herzberg, Mausner, and Synderman further developed the dual-factor theory of motivation (8). They described people as having two sets of needs: to avoid pain and to grow psychologically. To further illustrate this concept, motivational research was done with 200 engineers and accountants on feelings of satisfaction and whether these feelings affected personal relationships and well-being.

Although some researchers (9) believe that Maslow's and Herzberg's approaches to motivation theory cannot always be supported, both theorists have contributed much to the understanding of work motivation by concentrating attention on the importance of job content factors. Herzberg's research on job satisfaction substantiates the fact that motivation to work is based on the satisfaction of man's highest order of needs.

McGREGOR'S THEORY X AND THEORY Y

Douglas McGregor has classified traditional management theories as Theory X (10). Some of the beliefs he holds result from this logic: People will avoid work, if possible, because they dislike it; therefore, most people must be controlled, directed, coerced, and threatened. This theory assumes people want direction, have little ambition, avoid responsibility, yet want security. Managers who ascribe to this theory use fear and threats to motivate personnel.

They supervise closely, delegate little responsibility, and do not consider personal participation in planning. People behave by not accepting responsibility and challenge because of what the system has done to them, not because of their inherent nature. McGregor believes that as long as management strategies are based on Theory X, managers will be unable to discover and fully use potentials of their personnel (5, p. 62).

Theory Y, a newer development in management as classified by

McGregor, presents the following assumptions: People like work and really enjoy it; they are self-directed and seek responsibility; and most people have imagination, creativity, ingenuity, and other intellectual capacities that are only partly used (5, p. 62). Theory-Y managers freely use positive incentives (like praise and recognition and providing opportunities for individual growth), delegate responsibilities, and encourage participation in problem solving.

McGregor's Theory Y has implications for nurse-managers and can be seen as the basis for development of a positive work atmosphere that would motivate staff members to work to their full potential.

LIKERT'S THEORY

Recent research shows that the correlation between morale and productivity is nonexistent. There can be high morale with low productivity and low morale with high productivity (4, p. 152). Morale is one of the factors Rensis Likert tested. He defined it as "the total satisfaction a person derives from his job, his work group, his boss, the organization, and the environment" (11). Other characteristics, such as the personality of the individual and feelings of satisfaction, play an integral part in morale. Likert equates morale and productivity for complex and varied work as moderately high. When the job performance is dependent upon an individual worker on the team, the workers who like their job are more likely to be motivated to produce (4, p. 152).

Other contributions made by Likert are related to the manager's attitude toward his subordinates. Likert believes that, if the manager is to be effective, he is highly oriented toward his subordinates, uses communications to keep his team working together as a whole, and encourages and fosters supportive relationships among all group members (11, p. 70). This he terms the *participative management theory*. An ideal way to motivate staff members would be to provide some way for need satisfaction through the job itself. If the environment were conducive to openness, trust, and support from management, members of a nursing team would tend to have reason to be motivated.

OTHER MOTIVATION THEORIES

Other researchers and writers have contributed much to the study of human motivation, and the reader is directed to the bibliography for further reading in motivational theories. A brief listing of theories will be given here.

- Victor Vroom began the expectancy model of motivation in the 1960s in his description of force as motivation (12). *Expectancy* refers to the extent that the person feels his efforts will lead to first-level performance outcome.
- Luthans builds upon the Vroom model and suggests that Vroom's model could be used in addition to measuring a worker's output. With this in mind, managers could determine how important various personal goals are (13).
- Smith and Cranny's expectancy model promotes an understanding of the process of motivation by working with the human behavioral approach. A three-way relationship between effort (motivation), satisfaction, and reward is explored. Only effort (motivation) actually affects performance (14).
- McClelland, a Harvard psychologist, has also investigated achievement motive in people (15). His research has shown that achievement-oriented people will tend to translate their thinking into action and suggests that people who score high in achievement motivation are motivated by the interest in their work, love of success, and accomplishment (4, p. 151).
- The theory of behavior modification developed by Skinner describes types of reinforcement of motivation in humans (16). Positive reinforcement is most recommended since it increases the likelihood of a desired response. A simple nod of approval by a head nurse to a staff nurse is significant in the motivation of that employee.
- S. W. Gellerman has written management theories describing three methods that positively motivate (17). Stretching (increasing difficulty level), management by objectives (giving broad directions to encourage goal achievement), and participation (including staff's comments before making decisions about their work) are methods that are workable in motivating staff to improve performance.

APPLICATION OF MOTIVATION THEORY

The present writings on motivation theory do not allow us to say completely what motivates people or how the phenomenon takes place. Theories can always be challenged, expanded, and discarded, yet the nurse-manager in a health care facility is still faced with the day-to-day operational need to motivate employees.

From the empirical evidence that has been collected, it appears that the best motivator is a challenging job that allows a feeling of achievement, responsibility, growth, advancement, enjoyment of the work itself, and earned recognition — especially with professional people and highly skilled workers such as nurses.

One of the greatest challenges in motivation is developing the ability in the manager to help his workers really understand their complex needs and to help satisfy these ever-changing needs within the organization.

BEHAVIORAL CONSIDERATIONS

People have been getting others to perform tasks ever since the beginning of time. Methods have changed over the years from *forcing* techniques to *motivating* ones.

Motivation is defined as "the ability to get a person to do what you want him to do when you want it done, in a way you want it done and because he wants to do it" (18).

To motivate effectively, a person in the position to do so must discover something in each subordinate that:

- arouses his desires
- energizes his will
- serves as a basis for action or thought

Without this, the subordinate loses his sense of forward drive, and he runs out of energy.

Motivation is not a simple concept to either understand or implement. Current thinking suggests that motivated behavior is goal-directed behavior. A special process is involved. Figure 8-2 shows that a need is felt and defined by a person to reach a goal. Activity in the form of a behavioral response is attempted by the person feeling the need to relieve the same need. If this goal is blocked, the person becomes frustrated, and the original goal is not reached. If needs remain unsatisfied, another round of the process is initiated. If the goal is reached and the need satisfied, the person redefines her need in light of what she has learned.

Human behavior, in general, is motivated by this need-satisfying model. For example, people who need power will enter a field of administration or politics. Those who desire status may buy their way into a prestigious organization. People who fear threats to self-esteem avoid situations where intellectual competence is compromised.

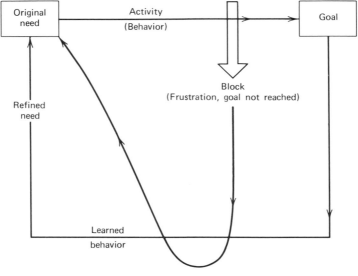

Figure 8-2.

Motivation refers to a way in which a need, urge, aspiration, or desire controls and directs as well as explains behavior in humans. A problem can occur in need satisfaction. As can be seen in Figure 8-2, people are not always able to satisfy their needs. As managers, nurses should be aware of the kinds of behaviors unsatisfied needs can elicit in staff members.

Frustration is a feeling that arises when blocks seem insurmountable and when failure to surmount them threatens a person's well-being. Frustration can occur when staff members have a strong need for esteem but the job is such that they cannot satisfy this need. Ideally, management might restructure the job so that personal needs for esteem could be met.

Once frustration of a blocked need occurs, a nurse-manager may notice one or several of the following recurrent defensive behaviors at work in the staff member:

1. *Aggression.* Aggression may be an outward attack toward a person or an obstacle or an inward attack toward the self. Behavior may be subtle (a scowl) or overt (actual physical attack). Aggression offers temporary relief to frustrated goal satisfaction but usually results in tension and negative human relationships.

2. *Withdrawal.* Withdrawal is a type of behavior in which the person physically or emotionally leaves the scene and may become apa-

thetic—for example, the person takes frequent sick days because he/she cannot handle the anxiety related to the job. The final solution is to quit the job. Withdrawal can be very detrimental to the unit staff as well as to the affected employee.

3. *Displacement.* Displacement is aggressive behavior directed to another person, such as a spouse, child, or peer. The target of the anger (e.g., the manager) and source of frustration is not the recipient of the aggressive actions, however.

4. *Compensation.* Compensation is a process by which a person makes up for a deficiency in his image of himself by strongly emphasizing some other feature that he regards as an asset. For example, the staff member with the blocked or frustrated need tends to engage actively in some other area of activity to make up for the deficiencies in the expected task. The compensation process is not necessarily related to the nursing tasks required.

5. *Repression.* In repression, the high level of energy and anxiety generated by the frustrated need satisfaction causes the person to lose awareness of the need. The need remains far from conscious awareness and is, in a sense, blocked out or denied.

6. *Regression.* Regression is a retreat in the face of stress to a behavior characteristic of an earlier level of development. In order to handle the pain and discomfort of the frustration, the person resorts to child-like behavior and horseplay when in the work situation in which the need must be met.

7. *Rationalization.* Rationalization is offering a socially acceptable explanation to justify or make acceptable otherwise unacceptable impulses, feelings, behaviors, and motives. For example, the worker convinces himself that the reason for not satisfying the need lies outside the self. This becomes less of an ego-deflating device than the real reason.

THE DEVELOPMENT OF MOTIVATION IN THE NURSE-MANAGER

Nurses in the health care setting are in a position to use motivational techniques with any people who work under them. The nurse-manager (supervisor, head nurse, or team leader) can increase her ability to lead others if she uses positive motivational techniques. Nurse-managers who use positive motivational styles will emphasize positive reinforcement mechanisms. For example, the head nurse who comments on a staff member's excellent nursing care to the emphysema patient in room 622 or recommends a pay increase for the same employee because of her constant high-quality nursing care is using a positive motivation technique. Other positive styles include providing positive and frequent feedback and a simple "thank you" to a colleague for the work performed that day. It really does not take much effort to develop this approach.

Negative motivational styles are also being used by nurse-managers and can produce acceptable performers in many situations. There are penalties in the use of this negative approach, however, as unpleasant side effects can be produced by the negative style of leadership. In this manner, nurse-managers state directives with a threat or fear orientation always present — even to the possible dismissal of the worker. The goal is to frighten the staff member into doing a better job. Employees spend much of their time, consequently, hiding from or protecting themselves from the nurse-manager. As a result, much energy is wasted by the employees as they try to cover their tracks or use scape-goating, blaming, or denial behavior with other workers.

Nurse-managers will tend, over time, to use one motivational style over the other one. The more predominant one will establish the overall attitude of nursing staff members on the unit and an expectancy of the behavior of the nurse-manager. The behavior of the nurse-manager will dictate the resulting group behavior in the staff.

SPECIFIC TECHNIQUES

In order to motivate staff on a unit, a conducive atmosphere must be established. Motivation is derived from motive or "the inner state that energizes, activates or moves and that directs or channels behavior toward goals" (19). Each person with the basic human needs identified by Maslow wants need satisfaction. In the work situation, managers set such conditions that may or may not satisfy these needs.

Behaviorists in management stress the concept that motivation of employees can be simply allowing them to influence their working environment by having a say in the decision-making process (20).

The nurse-manager can do other things to motivate her workers.

1. *Determine the objectives and purposes of the work to be done.* To motivate, it is necessary to know what you are trying to get someone to do.

2. *Integrate the needs and wants of the staff member with the inter-*

ests of the health care facility, including its goals and objectives. Allow staff members verbally to define their personal goals and to begin to work toward these goals.

3. *Communicate effectively with staff members so they have an effective role model.* Effective communication is one of the most difficult managerial tasks; messages from management are often misinterpreted by staff members. The nurse-manager should know which motivators work best with each employee and try to communicate an understanding of what she is doing to motivate that employee. Listen with undivided attention to each employee.

4. *Empathize with subordinates and try to see and feel the situation as the staff member does.* Unless the nurse-manager can do this, motivation efforts are going to be casual ones based solely on salary—the traditional motivator.

5. *Remove traditional blocks between the employee and the work to be done.* Lack of preparation and poor equipment, facilities, and work conditions should not interfere with the process of motivation and should be eliminated before a staff member can be motivated to perform effectively.

6. *Develop teamwork among staff members.* Integrate each employee's need satisfaction with that of other employees to lead to a coordinated group effort. Keep style positive with all members. A negative motivational approach for any staff person discourages total teamwork. Do not belittle a staff member. Do not criticize a member in front of others. Try not to play favorites or make exceptions because you like one staff person more than another. Other staff will resent this and become unmotivated. The nurse-manager should think of employees as a group and do what is best for the entire group. Through careful thought and planning, the nurse-manager can provide much individual employee motivation that will make the entire group more effective.

7. *Be an effective decision maker.* The quality of being wishy-washy shows lack of confidence, self-esteem, and determination. Staff will react by lacking confidence in the nurse-manager.

8. *Recognize you own biases and prejudgments so you can remain objective.* Keep staff members informed of their performance and allow them to know about changes that may affect them.

9. *Remember that staff development is a necessary part of motivation.* As a nurse-manager, go out of your way to enable staff members to develop and grow educationally and as people. Take responsibility for the growth and action of your staff. Encourage independence by allowing staff to solve problems, show initiative, and think creatively.

10. *Learn from others and from the ideas, suggestions, and problem solutions that are brought to you as a nurse-manager.* Encourage freedom of expression in your staff. Allow each member to make her own job interesting as long as goals and objectives are attained. Use tact and courteousness in interaction.

11. *Be aware that motivation lies within each person.* Your role as nurse-manager is to cultivate and release the forces already present in each staff person. You can direct into productive channels each of the goals staff members want and need. Some people are able to achieve some self-realization, but most people do not. Be aware that others do strive for self-realization and, as a nurse-manager, encourage each staff member to move upward on the stairway to self-realization by motivating that person. Look for opportunities to encourage the staff member by providing incentives to fulfill her needs and wants. Provide her with ways to achieve work satisfaction. Give the staff member responsibility and opportunity for achievement. Use each person's valuable resources to plan and implement effective patient care.

12. *Encourage involvement by staff members in the decision-making process.* This helps to increase productivity and then enhances the quality of nursing care given to patients. A good vehicle for the implementation of this process is the team conference. The development of trust between the nurse-manager and staff members is a necessary first step in allowing freedom for the decision-making process. Involvement by unit members increases interaction among members of the group, increases acceptance of members, and permits them to exercise more influence on the environment through suggestions and ideas. In addition, workers have the opportunity to assume responsibility for aiding management in tackling problems and identifying viable solutions. If staff are not involved, they may develop varying negative adaptive behaviors as well as feelings of powerlessness and apathy, as they have no influence on what is happening.

Increasing an employee's influence and involvement can help increase productivity and morale and, as a result, improve the quality of nursing care. This is a motivational strategy that all nurse-managers should endeavor to achieve.

13. *Consult with colleagues and seek advice on a formal basis as well as on an informal one.* This helps to achieve a feeling of joint responsibility in the organization. Nurse-managers can provide an environment to motivate staff if a consultative attitude and atmosphere is encouraged.

Through the use of these techniques and suggestions, a nurse-manager may begin to develop in a staff a high degree of motivation to improve output and increase the quality of nursing care administered.

In working with staff and clients in the health care setting, it becomes necessary for nurse-managers to be aware of work effectiveness and its ramifications. Understanding human behavior is essential in improving job performance of the staff on particular units so quality health care will result. Factors such as money, security, and status as well as the more involved competence, power, and achievement play an important role in work motivation. The works of many theorists are taken under consideration when planning ways to motivate a group of people with a common goal. It is helpful for the nurse-manager to have a working knowledge of theories described in this chapter in order to plan and implement patient care objectives. The modern nurse-manager helps each person develop his or her own talents and attempts to keep a close relationship between objectives and goals of the organization and individual needs requiring some degree of satisfaction in her

REFERENCES

1. Alexander E: *Nursing Administration,* ed 2. St Louis, The CV Mosby Co, 1978, p. 100.
2. Taylor F: *Shop Management.* New York, Harper, 1919, p. 113.
3. Maslow AH: *Motivation and Personality,* ed 2. New York, Harper & Row, 1970, p. 53.
4. Beyers M, Phillips C: *Nursing Management for Patient Care.* Boston, Little Brown & Co, 1979, p. 146.
5. Marriner A: Motivation of personnel. *Supervisor Nurse* 7:60, October 1976.
6. Maslow AH: *Toward a Psychology of Being.* Princeton, NJ, Van Nostrand, 1968, pp. 153–154, 160–165.
7. Herzberg F: One more time: how do you motivate employees? *Harvard Bus Rev* 46:91, 1973.
8. Herzberg F, et al: *The Motivation to Work.* New York, John Wiley & Sons Inc, 1960, p. 101.
9. Strauss G, Sayler L: *Personnel: The Human Problems of Management.* Englewood Cliffs, NJ, Prentice-Hall, 1967, p. 136.
10. McGregor D: *The Human Side of Enterprise.* New York, McGraw-Hill Book Co, 1960, p. 42.
11. Likert R: *New Patterns of Management.* New York, McGraw-Hill Book Co, 1961, p. 15.
12. Vroom V: *Work and Motivation.* New York, John Wiley & Sons Inc, 1966, p. 2.
13. Luthans F: *Introduction to Management: A Contingency Approach.* New York, McGraw-Hill Book Co, 1976, p. 25.
14. Smith FP, Cranny CJ: Psychology of men at work. *Ann Rev Psychology* 19:469, 1968.

15. McClelland D: *The Achieving Society.* Princeton, NJ, Van Nostrand, 1961, p. 26.
16. Skinner BF: Where Skinner's theories work. *Bus Week* Dec. 2, 1972, p. 64.
17. Gellerman S: *Motivation and Productivity.* New York, Am Management Association, 1963, p. 105.
18. *Motivation.* Trainaides Filmstrip—Supervision and Management. Glendale, Calif, Trainaide Educational Systems, American Hospital Supply Corp, 1970.
19. Berelson B, Steiner G: *Human Behavior—An Inventory of Scientific Findings.* New York, Harcourt Brace & World, 1964, p. 246.
20. Stevens E: *Management and Leadership in Nursing.* New York, McGraw-Hill Book Co, 1978, p. 155.

BIBLIOGRAPHY

Periodicals

Allen R: Turning a staff into a team. *Nursing '75* 5:91–92, March 1975.
Axne S, et al: Staff motivation through a self help design. *Supervisor Nurse* 7:65, October 1976.
Fleming AS: Motivating a staff plagued by failures. *Nursing '75* 5:86–88, March 1975.
Ganong W, Ganong J: Motivation, Maslow and me. *Supervisor Nurse* 4:25–32, July 1973.
Gunderson, K, Percy S, Canedy B, et al: How to control professional frustration. *Am J Nurs* 77:1180, July 1977.
Herzberg F: One more time: how do you motivate employees? *Harvard Bus Rev* 46:53, January-February 1968.
Lasea S: Motivation, evaluation and leadership. *J Nurs Adm* 2:17, September-October 1978.
Mager R, Pipe P: You really oughta wanna or how not to motivate people. *Nursing '76* 6:65, August 1976.
Marriner A: Motivation of personnel. *Supervisor Nurse* 7:60, October 1976.
Nusinoff JR: How to motivate your employees toward more effective patient care. *Hospital Topics* 54:50, March-April 1976.
Roche WJ, MacKinnon NL, Motivating people with meaningful work. *Harvard Bus Rev* 48:97, May-June 1970.
Skinner BF: Where Skinner's theories work. *Bus Week,* pp. 64–65, Dec. 2, 1972.
Smith FP, Cranny CJ: Psychology of men at work. *Ann Rev Psychology* 19:469–477, 1968.
Ulrich RA: Herzberg revisited: factors in job dissatisfaction. *J Nurs Adm* 8:19–24, October 1978.

Books

Alexander E: *Nursing Administration in the Hospital Health Care System.* St Louis, The CV Mosby Co, 1978, p. 100.

Berelson B, Steiner G: *Human Behavior — An Inventory of Scientific Findings.* New York, Harcourt Brace & World, 1964, p. 246.

Beyers M, Phillips C: *Nursing Management for Patient Care.* Boston, Little Brown & Co, 1979.

Ganong JM, Ganong WL: *Nursing Management Concepts, Functions, Techniques and Skills.* Germantown, Md, Aspen System Corp, 1976, pp. 177–201.

Gellerman SW: *Motivation and Productivity.* New York, Am Management Association, 1963, pp. 105–121.

Herzberg F: *Work and the Nature of Man.* Cleveland, World Publishing Co, 1973, pp. 99–111.

Herzberg F, et al: *The Motivation to Work.* New York, John Wiley & Sons Inc, 1960.

Likert R: *New Patterns of Management.* New York, McGraw-Hill Book Co, 1961.

Luthans F: *Introduction to Management: A Contingency Approach.* New York, McGraw-Hill Book Co, 1976.

Maslow AH: *Toward a Psychology of Being,* ed 2. Princeton, NJ, Van Nostrand, 1968, p. 42.

Maslow AH (ed): *Motivation and Personality,* ed 2. New York, Harper & Row, 1970, pp. 35–58.

McClelland D: *The Achieving Society.* Princeton, NJ, Van Nostrand, 1961, pp. 36–62.

McGregor D: *The Human Side of Enterprise.* New York, McGraw-Hill Book Co, 1960.

Stevens E: *Management and Leadership in Nursing.* New York, McGraw-Hill Book Co, 1978, pp. 127–128, 139, 154–155, 159.

Strauss G, Sayler L: *Personnel: The Human Problems of Management.* Englewood Cliffs, NJ, Prentice-Hall, 1967.

Taylor FW: *Shop Management.* New York, Harper Brothers, 1919.

Vroom V: *Work and Motivation.* John Wiley & Sons Inc, 1966.

Yura H, Ozimek D, Walsh, M: *Nursing Leadership Theory and Process.* New York, Appleton-Century-Crofts, 1976, pp. 114–115, 161, 171–172, 177.

Yura H, Walsh MB: *The Nursing Process,* ed 3. New York, Appleton-Century-Crofts, 1978, pp. 51, 77–86.

Filmstrip

Motivation. Trainaides Filmstrip — Supervision and Management. Glendale, Calif. Trainaide Educational Systems, American Hospital Supply Corp, 1970.

9. Staffing and Staffing Patterns

"A Jigsaw Puzzle"

Joyce L. Schweiger, R.N., M.S.

BEHAVIORAL OBJECTIVES

After reviewing this chapter, the reader will be able to

- describe the interrelationship between the health care agency's philosophy of nursing and its staffing patterns
- construct a staffing pattern that will enable the staff to provide quality patient care
- identify the value of a pilot study in developing a basic staffing pattern within a health care agency
- identify the variables, expected or unexpected, that contribute to the complexity of staffing within a health care agency

One of the most significant and critical factors that has affected quality care delivery today is staffing. The problems of providing the appropriate number and levels of care providers to facilitate patient care have in some instances proved to be seemingly unsolvable. This does not imply that those responsible for providing the care are not interested in the welfare of the patient and have not and are not continuing to meet the demands for increase in the number of care providers. There is much more involved with the staffing question than is usually considered unless one is faced with the ongoing dilemma. The complexity of staffing evolves from expected or unexpected extraneous variables. In order for nurses to understand and to be able to cope with the staffing dilemma, it is important to identify the variables and what effect they have on the problem. The following list comprises

those variables that are seen as influencing factors on efforts to attain
appropriate staffing:

- cost
- federal government
- agency philosophy
- patient assignments
- work schedules
- fringe benefits
- type and location of facility
- availability of care providers
- length of stay
- nursing leadership

No single variable listed can be considered more important than
another. Therefore, it is important that each item is singularly
reviewed.

COST

As was indicated in Chapter 3, the spiraling cost of health care delivery has been phenomenal. The cost of running a health care agency
has taken its toll on the working budget of the agencies. The rising cost
in equipment, expendable supplies, and general overhead has forced
administrators critically to assess the staffing budget. It is no longer
sufficient for a nursing administrator to request an increase in staffing
budget based on day-to-day census and number of personnel available
to provide care. Justification is needed to increase allocations in this
area of the budget. The nursing administrator must employ a method
of patient classification in order to justify requests. If requests are not
appropriately justified, it is not uncommon for the agency administrator to consult with an industrial engineering firm to conduct time and
motion studies. This is a very basic, realistic approach to determine
the number of staff needed to perform specific tasks. However, it is a
method that does not measure needs, behavior, and reactions of the
patient and the care providers. Needless to say, this cost-saving approach is appealing to the financial committee of the agency, but the
result is usually unsatisfactory in regard to total patient care.

It is difficult to try to compromise cost and quality care. For example,
primary nursing is seen as the answer to individualized holistic care. It

is also seen as a way to bring professionals back to the bedside, where their expertise is needed. Hospital administrators respond to this idea in a similar fashion. They think "Great idea, care will certainly be improved, but — ." But what do they do with all the nonprofessionals? And who is going to pay the high salaries and benefits of a staff that is almost entirely composed of professionals? Again, for the administrator, cost surfaces as the inevitable barrier. However, Marram (1) found that primary nurses tend to receive fewer instances of overtime and sickness that tend in the long run to be costly items.

One answer to the staffing dilemma is small-scale planning. This involves implementation of a concept — in this instance, primary nursing — on one unit as a pilot study in order to gather data to substantiate care needs and cost before a decision is made. It is unwise to disrupt the entire structure of an agency. A small-scale plan, with ample time for evaluation — whether it is with a patient classification program, time and motion studies, or a pilot primary nursing study — can result in a carefully controlled analysis of accumulated data that will result in containment of the cost variable.

FEDERAL GOVERNMENT

Federal regulations concerning audit and review requirements for medical care have now expanded to encompass nursing. The amendments (1972) to Title XI of the Social Security Act created Professional Standards Review Organizations (PSROs) charged with reviewing Social Security-funded health care with respect to medical necessity, quality of care, and whether care was given at the level most economic for patients' needs (2). The impact of these regulations has been felt by nursing.

According to Somers (3), if the concept of federal review is not reckoned with in an appropriate manner, the movement will be away from the present catchall criteria for nursing care toward concurrent justification of every nursing task — justification derived from a comparative audit of actual nursing tasks to specific criteria by diagnosis with reimbursement by task. Somers believes that this action would hold grave implication for nursing service and staffing in particular. It would hamper critical thinking and remove creativity from nursing.

Close regulation of activities as stipulated by federal legislation will not allow flexibility, which is an important component in providing patient care. Rigid task analysis reinforces the cost variable but does not improve care. The answers can be, and have been, in many instances, found within the nursing services. An example of this is the nursing audit. Whether concurrent or retrospective, the audit does provide data that aid in determining the number and type of staff necessary to provide quality care without outside monitoring.

AGENCY PHILOSOPHY

Before any attempts can be made to develop a staffing pattern within a health care agency, it is essential that the agency has a working philosophy. It is assumed that all health care agencies have a philosophy, but it is not always a working one. This philosophy is the base from which the quality of nursing care practice evolves.

Agency philosophy varies in accordance with whom the agency serves, where it serves, and why it serves. As a result, staffing will be firmly entrenched in the matrix of the society that the agency serves. The staffing pattern in a public health agency must be designed and tailored to meet the specific needs of that particular community (4). Since communities today are in a constant state of flux, the philosophy of both the agency and nursing department must, at times, be altered to meet changing needs. These alterations in turn affect the staffing pattern. An agency that has either internal or external responsibilities for providing patient care must have a workable philosophy at its grassroots.

PATIENT ASSIGNMENTS

Over the past three decades there has been a great deal of vacillation in nursing in regard to patient assignment. This vacillation primarily concerns the method of patient assignment used within a hospital or extended care facility to provide the patient with optimum care. Those who are responsible for deciding patient assignment methods must consider the type of patient in the unit; the number of available professional and nonprofessional staff; the type of facility—long-term or acute care, specialty or general; the care providers' qualifications to uphold the nursing philosophy; and the length of stay for the patient. These are major considerations in selecting the most efficient and effective patient assignment method. The success or failure of both the flow of work and its quality frequently depends upon the method of assignment.

Four major types of patient assignment have evolved over the past three decades: case, functional, team, and primary nursing. Each was developed at a critical time in nursing and for specific reasons based on social, economic, or political events. *Case* nursing has a history that dates back to the beginning of the century, when nurses were hired by families to provide for a patient's special needs that the families were unable to meet. This type of patient assignment lingers today in the concept of private duty nursing. It is also reflected in intensive or critical care units where, if feasible, one nurse is assigned to no more than two patients.

The *functional* method of assigning, which is a task-oriented method of providing minimal to adequate patient care, is used more often than not in care settings. The functional method is considered a less expensive method of providing care than the other three methods. The tasks are divided among the staff, and the input of the professional nurse usually encompasses the dispensing of medications and the supervision of work. The concept of holistic care is overlooked. Fragmentation of care most suitably describes this method of assignment. Unfortunately, it is the method used if staff is either unavailable or poorly distributed. It also removes the burden of accountability from those involved in care and places it totally with the nurse-in-charge. The only positive note about the functional assignment method is cost containment. This method appears to be less costly.

The *team* nursing method is used in many facilities. This method is presented exceptionally well by Kron (5), who described team nursing not as a procedure but as the implementation of a philosophy that states that a group of people led by a knowledgeable nurse who makes use of everyone's capabilities can effectively meet the nursing needs of a group of patients. However, the method is rarely used as she describes it. Instead, many times the team leader finds herself dispensing medications or in some instances giving care to seriously ill patients. The time that should be spent supervising, directing, assessing, assisting, and teaching team members and patients is rarely allocated. In this instance, the team concept resembles the functional method but is given a different title.

The method of *primary* nursing assignment seems to be the answer to all the patients' needs. In primary nursing, a nurse is assigned to provide total care on a 24-hour basis to a select number of patients from time of admission through discharge (5). Some administrators find this method controversial. Their first reaction is that it is too costly because too many professionals are needed. Many administrators do not want to recognize that an increase in professional staff who have more expertise will shorten patient stay, improve the quality of care, enhance the bonds of communication among professionals, and attain the goal of holistic care that includes the physician, the nurse, and the patient and his family. As nurses, we have not articulated and demonstrated these outcomes.

WORK SCHEDULES

The person who is responsible for the selection of a method of care assignment frequently finds the complexity of selecting the method further complicated by the fifth variable—work schedules. At one time, scheduling was relatively simple; in fact, most head nurses were responsible for planning their own staff's schedule and submitting a copy of it to nursing administration approximately two to four weeks before it is posted. Now, scheduling has become a major chore and is frequently placed in the hands of a staffing secretary or staffing supervisor. In addition to the effects of overlapping variables that affect staffing already discussed, other issues play a significant role. Many of the issues will be familiar because they occur no matter what the type or size of the agency. Specific logistical difficulties in scheduling are related to staff members' family responsibilities and desires for specific days off; shift rotation, leaves of absence; vacation desires (specific time to coincide with mates); numbers, preparation, and expertise of float staff; job tension (i.e., special stresses of intensive care nursing); need for head nurse to relieve the nursing office staff on weekends; absence of supervisors in agency; ward managers or ward secretaries off on weekends with no replacement; ward secretary under the umbrella of medical administration, not nursing. These issues must be considered and accommodated by the person responsible for staffing and must, therefore, be given careful thought in scheduling.

FRINGE BENEFITS

Who will work for what today? Pick up the newspaper, listen to media. There is always a faction somewhere in the health care system that is unhappy with the status quo. Many times the reasons may be justifiable; other times they seem to be based on trifles. Pension plans, insurance policies, annual accumulative sick time, yearly physicals, dental and eye examinations are all part of the benefit package that the employee is desiring and receiving today. These are but a few of the requests and demands. All of the above factors must be built into budgets and are costly endeavors for the health care agencies. Therefore, in order to keep those already employed personnel reasonably satisfied, it may be necessary to make a sacrifice in another area, such as not hiring additional staff. Fringe benefits weigh heavily on staffing, as they directly affect the implementation of the agency's philosophy.

TYPE AND LOCATION OF FACILITY

The type of the facility also has a direct bearing on staffing and staffing patterns. For example, one must consider whether the agency is general or specific in type. Does it include specialty areas such as high-risk nursery, burn center, or hemodialysis unit? Does it have outpatient services housed within the facility? Does it have satellite programs, a viable emergency room, or a rehabilitation unit? If it is a specialty agency, does it provide day care or night care or both? Is it a small facility with 20 patients or a larger facility with 100 or more patients? Is it considered a therapeutic center or a custodial center that encompasses a therapeutic component? Is it a long-term care center that includes therapeutic, restorative, rehabilitative, or custodial care? This information will again affect the staffing component (6).

In addition to the type of facility, the location of the facility cannot be overlooked. Accessibility of any agency will often determine its use, which inadvertently will affect staffing. A center-city hospital in a busy urban area will have different staffing needs than a 20 to 60 bed suburban facility that has access to a metropolitan multifaceted facility.

AVAILABILITY OF CARE PROVIDERS

What are the resources that are available to the agency to provide the care? Is the agency located in a city or town that has colleges, universities, or hospital-based nursing programs in close proximity so these can be used as sources for potential employees? Also the agency's philosophy must fulfill the needs of the potential employee.

The shortage of nurses has been investigated from the standpoint of those nurses who do not want to work rather than those nurses who are not available to work. In 1978 Seyboldt et al (7) presented the findings of a survey taken in a 310-bed university hospital in Salt Lake City, Utah, that revealed that the most compelling reason for disinterest in working and turnover in staff was a lack of motivation. To the majority of these nurses, there seemed to be no opportunity to grow, to learn new things, or to make independent decisions. Even though the primary motivation for professional development rests in the individual nurse, it is the responsibility of the hiring agency to provide other incentives. These incentives are in addition to the fringe benefits discussed previously. Incentives are necessary to attract and keep capable care providers. Motivation theories should not be confined to workshops but applied in practice. Motivation of people is a continuous process, and its presence is reflected in the attitudes and quality of care given by the staff.

Motivation of personnel begins at the top and goes down the line. If the leaders lack motivation, they cannot possibly provide incentives for those they oversee. It is a chain reaction. Techniques to use in motivation have been clearly identified and detailed in Chapter 8.

LENGTH OF EMPLOYMENT

The length of stay of employees is never predictable, and many of the reasons for their leaving are the same as or similar to those of the nurses who no longer desire to work—that is, working conditions, job dissatisfaction, and failure to provide an opportunity for growth. In addition, the process of hiring, the placement of personnel, and over-promising are other factors contributing to length of stay.

Hiring and placement problems can be overcome if the qualifications of the person applying, her amount of preparation and experience, and her interest/preference are considered. This effort is time-consuming, but is an essential part of the initial interview. If the right person is put into the right job and the right numbers of people are doing the job, the hiring and placement problems can be alleviated. If what the potential employee wants is not available at the time, but may be in the near future, say so. Do not promise or guarantee anything that cannot occur. If the person has the qualifications you are seeking, be honest. She will probably take the job and will be willing to wait for the opportunity for the position to open.

NURSING LEADERSHIP

The style of leadership is reflected in staff performance. A staff is only as effective as its leader. In staffing a nursing department, the nursing administrator should be a strong, decisive, well-organized, knowledgeable decision maker. She must be able to assess where nursing is, and where it is going in terms of goals in the agency before she can determine the number and distribution of staff. She must be certain that she reviews and examines the philosophy, the objectives, and the goals of the nursing department. These areas must be reflected in her decision about the number of staff needed and in her selection of the staffing pattern.

The variables that affect staffing and staffing patterns are numerous and varied. The variables that have been discussed can be added to by every reader, but they have been presented as a starting point, something to think about as she approaches the problem of staffing.

After the inevitable variables are accepted, the final step is to determine an appropriate staffing pattern. The availability of time to develop and activate a satisfactory staffing pattern is a major concern in nursing. Time is needed to decide which pattern is the most suitable for patient care and also acceptable to the staff. It would be relatively simple if one pattern would be satisfactory to all clinical areas, but this is frequently not possible. In order to determine the right staffing pattern, those responsible for the choice must have time to think, plan, present, and evaluate.

There are data needed before a staffing pattern can be determined. For example, some considerations are the size of unit, physical layout of the unit, accessibility of ancillary health care units, type of patient assigned to unit, percentage of occupancy in unit, plus the scheduling variables already discussed. After all of these factors are considered, a decision can be made about an appropriate staffing pattern that can be implemented in a pilot unit. The pilot unit should be small and the staff willing to participate in the project. This is a change, and any change, no matter how minor, should be fully and completely discussed with the involved staff to allow them verbal input. No matter what pattern is introduced, if the staff does not want it, it probably will not work. A new staffing pattern should be in effect for a trial period of at least six weeks. At the end of this period, a thorough evaluation of its apparent success or failure must be done. The evaluation should include written critiques, group and individual staff interviews, and a patient questionnaire survey related to care received. If the positive feedback outweighs the negative, the pattern can be considered for possible expansion into other units, but this can only be done if the pattern meets the needs of those units. Remember that what is effective in a specialty unit will usually not be appropriate for a general unit. Alterations can be made and the pilot pattern used as a framework.

Scheduling patterns to choose from vary: conventional; cyclical; 40 hours, 4 days; 7 days on, 7 days off; 12-hour plan; and team schedule are just a few. Each pattern has advantages and disadvantages that can only be determined by the agency needs, resources, and personnel policies.

Conventional staffing is the oldest pattern of staffing. The amount of staff needed to provide care is usually determined by either the head nurse or supervisor. Patterns are determined according to existing nursing policies. When patient care cannot be provided for by the number of existing staff who are assigned to a particular unit, the supervisors will be expected to provide additional help from other units or from a floating pool of nurses. When this conventional method is used, the pattern for staffing is usually determined by the head nurse during the day and evening tour and by the supervisor for the night tour of duty. This will vary from agency to agency. Use of the conventional method can cause a great deal of dissension among staff, since an existing obvious split in authority and loyalty is often reflected in the quality of care given and priorities set by staff members.

Cyclic patterns of staffing are patterns that repeat themselves. The amount of highly skilled professional time spent in scheduling functions is reduced. Other advantages cited in 1978 by Eusanio (8) are: the good and bad days off are spread equitably among all employees; schedules are known in advance by each employee; the scheduling of correct numbers and mixes of personnel on duty each day is simplified. Once the master schedule is developed, it can be repeated for each period (4, 6, 7, 12 weeks). Continuity of care is provided by minimizing floating. In this pattern, there is a constant number of people. The cyclical schedule also considers the number of float nurses, absenteeism, illnesses, vacation, and other variables, such as leave of absences.

The two methods, conventional and cyclic, described above are usually used when the component of working hours is distributed over 40 hours per week or 80 hours in a pay period, but they can be applied to changes within the framework. For example, perhaps the work situation in a particular unit would be conducive to 40 hours in a 4-day week. Several of the advantages to this were presented in a 1972 *RN* review (9): weekends off and overlapping shifts that would allow better coverage for mealtime and nursing care of long-term patients. The staff member would be working 16 days less per year, but the same number of hours with full pay. In addition, extra pay would be earned for the 9 to 10 hours each work day. Another schedule described could be 3 10-hour shifts in one week and 4 10-hour shifts the next, with every other weekend off. The shifts would be joined by the use of part-time personnel.

Another feasible staffing pattern described in 1974 by Cleveland and Hutchins (10) is the 7-day on, 7-day off work schedule. This pattern would be a 10-hour day with 7 days worked and 7 days off. It would be based upon two 24-hour working staffs rather than one. The staff member would be paid for 80 hours, but there would be no vacation or holiday time. An allowance of 70 hours would be assigned to sick time. Variations in this pattern could include a redistribution of the 70 hours set aside for sick time to allow time for vacation and holidays. This variation would depend upon the agency's philosophy and also upon the number of overall absentee days for illness in nursing service, within a specific framework of time. The positive aspects of the 7-day on, 7-day off pattern are: strong interpersonal relationships between patients and staff due to the number of consecutive days spent together; an increase in staff motivation in their anticipation of the consecutive 7 days off; and, most important, a decided improvement in the quality and continuity of patient care.

Another example of schedule patterns is the 12-hour plan. In 1976 Cales (11) described the pros and cons of this pattern. The 12-hour plan was introduced in a nursery unit on a 6-week schedule. Extensive preplanning was done. Briefly, in this pattern the work week began on Wednesday and ended the following Tuesday, then 7 days off. There were four units: two worked 7 A.M. to 7 P.M., two worked 7 P.M. to 7 A.M., alternating each week with each other and each had every other weekend included in their time off. The staff quota was three RNs, 1 LPN, 1 aide for each shift. The major plus was that the newborns were getting quality care; this could be attributed primarily to continuity of care. Each shift received the report from the same shift to which they had reported to twelve hours earlier. Some of the problems were: family problems of staff members, inservice programs that had to be scheduled more frequently and presented on the working shifts. Breaks were also encouraged to keep up the level of efficiency. Occasionally near the end of a work week there were personality clashes. However, despite the problems, the staff in the nursery felt that this pattern met their needs.

The last example of schedule patterns is less familiar — team staffing. This concept is well described in 1974 by Frobe (12). The team pattern is based on levels of experience and compatability of staff members. As it is described, the staff members are scheduled to work as a unit, rotating through particular units and receiving days off together. Teams are identified by letters, such as A, B, C. Schedules are structured one year ahead, so that staff can plan. Emergencies that arise are handled from within and, if a leave of absence (LOA) is needed, it is handled within the group. This idea has been implemented with air traffic controllers groups and could be applied to nursing if there were available staff to provide specific team groups. The commonalities that exist with nursing and air traffic groups are wide fluctuation of work load and peak time for work load. For example, more planes fly during the day and evening; usually more extensive patient care is given during the day and evening; less planned activity exists in both fields at night. The team pattern in nursing would have to consider the single work tour of duty; rotation from team to team; time posted by name, not number; individual team assignment; number of personnel; ratio of professionals to nonprofessionals. The success of this pattern is based upon stability in working assignment, constructive peer competition, acceptance of criticism, and open communication.

The success of our health care delivery system today depends upon the care provided for the patient. The care given, in essence, is reflected by the number and quality of care providers the agency employs. New approaches to staffing must be considered, as well as all of the variables that affect staffing, if we are going to be successful in our attempts to control the health care delivery system of the nation.

REFERENCES

1. Marram G: The comparative costs of operating a team and primary nursing unit. *J Nurs Adm* 6:23, May 1976.
2. Walton MH: Quality assurance in health care. *Quality Assurance Models for Nursing Education.* New York, National League for Nursing, 1976, p. 29.

3. Somers JB: Purpose and performance: a system analysis of nurse staffing. *J Nurs Adm* 7:4, February 1977.
4. Regnery G: Patient care needs—an index for community health staffing. *Nurs Adm* 2: Fall 1977.
5. Kron T: *The Management of Patient Care,* ed 4. Philadelphia, WB Saunders Co, 1976, p. 22.
6. Donovan HM: *Nursing Administration—Managing the Enterprise.* St Louis, The CV Mosby Co, 1975, p. 106.
7. Seyboldt JW, et al: Turn over among nurses: it can be managed. *J Nurs Adm* 8:4–9, September 1978.
8. Eusanio PL: Effective scheduling—the foundation for quality care. *J Nurs Adm* 8:13, January 1978.
9. Four day work week? Oh, those long weekends! *RN* 3:42–45, January 1971.
10. Cleveland R, Hutchins C: Seven days vacation every other week. *Hospitals* 48:81–85, 1974.
11. Cales AD: A twelve-hour schedule experiment. *Supervisor Nurse* 7:71, June 1976.
12. Frobe D: Scheduling: by team individually. *J Nurs Adm* 4(3): 34, May-June 1974.

BIBLIOGRAPHY

Periodicals

Clark LE: A model for effective nurse staffing patient care. *J Nurs Adm* 7:22, February 1977.

Des Ormeaux SP: Implementation of the C.A.S.H. patient classification. *Supervisor Nurse* 8:29, April 1977.

Donovan HM: Determining priorities of nursing care. *Nurs Outlook* 11:44, January 1963.

Eusanio PL: Effective scheduling—the foundation for quality care. *J Nurs Adm* 8:12–18, January 1978.

Ganong WL, et al: The 12-hour shift: better quality, lower cost. *J Nurs Adm* 6:17, February 1976.

Harris DH: Staffing requirements. *Hospitals* 44:64, April 16, 1970.

Latham J, Fagan J: Control of Christmas holiday census and staffing. *J Nurs Adm* 9:19, October 1979.

Longest BB: Job satisfaction for registered nurses in the hospital setting. *J Nurs Adm* 4:46–52, March 1974.

Marram G: The comparative cost of operating a team in primary nursing care. *J Nurs Adm* 6:21–24, May 1976.

McCarthy D, Schifalaqua MM: Primary nursing: its implementation and six month outcome. *J Nurs Adm* 8:29–33, May 1978.

McKinnon HA, Elikson L: C.A.R.E.: a four track professional nurse classification and performance evaluation system. *J Nurs Adm* 7:42, April 1977.

Norby RB, et al: A nurse staffing system based upon assignment difficulty. *J Nurs Adm* 7:2, November 1977.

O'Malley CC: Application of systems engineering in nursing. *Am J Nurs* 69:2155, 1969.

Pardee G: Classifying patients to predict staffing requirements. *Am J Nurs* 67:517, March 1968.

Somers JB: Purpose or performance: a system analysis of nurse staffing. *J Nurs Adm* 7:4, February 1977.

Tally R, Graham K: A block scheduling system. *J Nurs Adm* 5:39, November-December 1975.

Warsler ME: Cyclic work schedules and a non nurse coordinator of staffing. *J Nurs Adm* 3:45, November-December 1973.

Zegeer LJ: Calculating a nurse staffing budget for a 20-bed unit at 100% occupancy. *J Nurs Adm* 7:11–14, February 1977.

Books

Donovan HM: *Nursing Service Administration.* St Louis, The CV Mosby Co, 1975, pp. 110–124.

Price E: *Staffing for Patient Care.* New York, Springer Publishing Co Inc, 1976, pp. 82–92.

10. Job Descriptions

"Vital Statistics"

Joyce L. Schweiger, R.N., M.S.

BEHAVIORAL OBJECTIVES

After reviewing this chapter, the reader will be able to

- develop the job description to reflect the objectives of management
- use the job description as a resource in planning, staffing, work organization, scheduling, productivity, review, and reporting
- use the job description in recruitment, orientation, training problems, and performance standards
- compare and contrast the job description with other evaluation tools to identify the total role position of the employee

Hospitals and other health care agencies should have a well-defined program for evaluating their personnel. In order for the criteria for evaluation to be developed, a level of standards must be identified. These standards appear in each job description, which provides a clear, detailed account of the employee's function. The job description is the basic tool used by both the employee and employer in identifying specific areas of performance.

There are practical uses of the job description:

- It saves time in the clinical setting so that each activity does not have to be spelled out.
- It provides a tool to ascertain that the person is functioning at the expected level of performance.
- It establishes a rational basis for the salary structure, identifying

why one position pays more than another. For example, it clarifies why the supervisor may receive a higher salary than the head nurse and why an aide with three years of experience would receive more than a novice who must be prepared by the staff development department.

- It clarifies relationships between jobs to avoid overlapping and gaps in accountability and responsibility. For example, in reviewing the specific duties of the head nurse and the staff nurse, it should be quite evident where the staff nurse's responsibility stops and the head nurse's accountability continues.
- It helps each employee analyze the duties so that he will have a clear concept of the job and all it entails. Each employee should be aware of the overlapping of roles and where responsibilities are assumed without justification.
- It helps to define the organizational structure and clearly identifies its goals and objectives (1).

The job description is a necessary adjunct to the agency's organization chart. The position designated on the chart will be described in detail in terms of the accountability, responsibility, and authority the job encompasses. Note that accountability has been included as a basic component. In this way, the employer is attempting to build quality assurance in the employee's position. Job descriptions are particularly valuable in stating not only the employee's responsibility but to whom and for what he is accountable. If these two areas are not clearly defined, the quality and quantity of work the employee does may not be adequately judged. Swansburg defines a job description as "a contract, a written report that outlines activities, responsibilities, and conditions of the work assignment" (1, p. 211). It is a description of a job. It is not a description of a person. This is an important distinction. For example, let us suppose that you do not have an infection control nurse in your setting because, in the past, there was no need for this position. Infections seemed to occur rarely. If they did occur, they were considered nonhospital or surgical-expected, determined by the type of surgical procedure performed. This classification was either decided by the physician or based on the report of the pathologist, if he was given the opportunity to render an opinion or a report. Now, the standards of practice require that you, in nursing, create this position as a preventive control mechanism and to keep the standards of care at a quality level. In order to introduce this new position and to be certain it will be well accepted, your first consideration may be who will qualify. Who will best be able to relate effectively with nursing staff, convince the physicians, and pacify the administration—right? No—wrong. A job description is not built around a specific person. This is one of the golden rules of an effective administration. Personalities have a way of directly influencing functions and roles. Without recognizing it, you may tend to write the job description emphasizing all the positive attributes and minimizing any personal deficiencies. It is necessary to identify the role of the infection control nurse. You may have a specific person in mind, one who is well liked, knowledgeable, flexible, respected by physicians, and who does not make waves. This sounds right for the job? Wrong again. A major portion of this position is in the area of accountability. *Accountability* is not a new word but an all-encompassing one. In nursing, accountability is concerned with what was done as compared with what should have been done(2). It is a measure of the efficiency and productivity of a person as judged against professional or nursing standards.

With this in mind, the nurse who has been preselected for infection control nurse would not fit because she "doesn't make waves." There are probably going to be waves in this situation since a change is introduced and, although it is a mandatory one, that does not mean it will be well received. The personality-versus-proficiency factor is one example of the controversies that may arise in writing a new job description or in rewriting an active one.

There are two alternatives open to the person writing the description: inside consultation or outside consultation. No one has more knowledge about the functions, operation, responsibility, and accountability of a specific position than those who are actively involved in the work setting. Behind-the-desk planning and preparation may seemingly lend more objectivity in writing a job description; however, this is small compensation in exchange for the overall knowledge of the active situation and problems involved.

If inside consultation is not applicable or available to you, the second alternative should be considered—outside consultation. Outside consultants are paid by management not only to guide and advise in writing job descriptions but, in some instances, actually to write the entire job description. The objectivity may be there, but frequently refinement of the position must be done and details clarified by the active participants.

FORMATS FOR JOB DESCRIPTIONS

The formats for job descriptions vary but remain similar in content as seen in the following outline (1, pp. 211–213).

A. Job Title (Subject)
B. Job Summary
    1. General description
    2. Responsibility
    3. Accountability
    4. Specific duties
       a. Performance standards
    5. Special demands
       a. Mental
       b. Physical
C. Qualifications
D. Employment Variables
E. Working Environment

Job Title

The title of the job description differs according to the detailing of the content of the position and according to the professional jargon used in a particular institution.

Job Summary

Specific questions must be raised before and during the preparation of the job summary (1, p. 215).

1. What is the job description based on?
2. What does it include?
3. How does it detail the position?
4. Does it reflect what it should reflect?
5. Does it fit the job?
6. Is it needed?

Each of these questions must be answered in detail and must be weighed equally. An analysis of each question is imperative in order to assess the clarity, completeness, and conciseness of the document. A thoughtful assessment of each question will prevent loopholes and vagueness in the finished product.

1. *What is the job description based on?* The job description is based on:

- the philosophy of the health care agency and the nursing service within the job description.
- the recognition by nursing service of the standards of care in practice that have been established by the Congress for Nursing Practice of the American Nurses Association. Practical application of performance standards should be apparent in the job description in the delineation of responsibilities and specific duties.
- information from within the Social Security Amendment of 1972, Public Law 92–603, applies. It mandates the establishment of Professional Standards Review Organizations (PSROs). Specifically related to nursing is Section 73, which says: "review of care provided by non-physician health care practitioners should be performed by their peers" (3). Unless the function-responsibilities of the nurse are specifically delineated in the job description, this review process will be difficult to carry out. Other influences on the job description format are the State Nurse Practice Act, the state licensure regulations for hospital and, in some instances, the JCAH criteria.

2. *What does the job description include?* The job description

- gives the position a title: head nurse, staff nurse, and so on.
- summarizes the basic functions of the position. The summary is a brief statement not more than one or two paragraphs long. It includes a general overview of the job functions. The scope of the position is encompassed in the title and job summary.
- delineates the duties and responsibilities of the position in detail under "Specific duties" and "Performance standards." In these areas, the criteria for performance evaluation should be readily identified, and it is strongly emphasized that, at this point, the employer should include a statement related to accountability.

3. *How does the job description detail the position?* The position is described fully. In addition to particular duties, the job description clearly indicates special demands, both mental and physical, that may be made of the employee in the job situation. There should be no doubt in the employee's mind about the expectations of performance after he has read the job description. The clarity and consiseness with which it

is written should provide the employee with a tool to use in his own self-evaluation of performance.

4. *What does the job description reflect?* Does the job description reflect the philosophy of nursing in the health care agency? Does it simulate the projected objectives and goals of the department? Is it simply task-oriented? The answers to these questions will provide insight into the conceptual framework of the nursing service.

5. *Does the description fit the job?* In the final analysis, does the job description actually say what that position encompasses? Is the scope of the job broad enough to allow a degree of generalization, yet specific enough to maintain its area of specialization?

6. *Is the job needed?* Is the job description simply a restatement of another job with just a change in title? Is it a position that has been created without any definite criteria or substantial evidence for the need? Frequently we find ourselves creating additional positions that may, after closer scrutiny, be unnecessary.

When you have answered these six questions, you will have completed the job summary as delineated in the outline presented earlier in this chapter. You are now ready to detail qualifications, employment variables, and the working environment.

Qualifications

There is a great deal of controversy about the level of preparation for a qualified nurse. Basic qualifications for a nurse are that she be (1) a graduate of a preservice-accredited educational program in nursing and (2) a nurse currently registered in the state in which she plans to practice.

The problem that arises with qualifications is twofold. The first part of the problem is related to salary, the second part to the nurse's professional status. For example, in certain areas of the United States, the diploma graduate and baccalaureate graduate are considered professional while the associate degree nurse is categorized, along with the licensed practical nurse, as a technical person. In addition, many hospitals do not offer a pay scale that is based on a level of preparation. This means that the nurse with baccalaureate preparation has the same base salary as the diploma or associate degree nurse. The discrepancy in pay scale can be a very delicate issue, and it is advisable that employers be explicit and definitive about this sensitive area when the job description is reviewed with the potential employee. If the situation demands, it would be advisable to justify the differences, if they exist, by example of level of performance. This is done to avoid confusion and subsequent dissatisfaction on the employee's part.

The second area related to qualifications concerns training and experience. Although it is often used, the term *training* should be deleted from the professional job description and replaced with *level of preparation*. The concern is to identify the minimal educational preparation by the applicant in order to be considered for the position designated and responsibilities described.

Job knowledge refers to the amount of academic preparation required for the position—for example, the depth of preparation it includes in the basic sciences, humanities, principles of nursing management, and leadership included in the nursing curriculum. What the employer is looking for in the individual's credentials will depend upon the position he wishes to fill.

Employment Variables

Employment variables are the hours and shifts the employee is required to work. If shift rotation is required, it will be noted here. Weekend work will be clarified, and also specific number of holidays required to work will be listed, either by name or number per year. All of these variables are subject to change by the employer more than any other as a result of changes in administrative philosophy and objectives, hospital policy, or labor-relation negotiations.

Working Environment

Under no circumstances can the working environment be vaguely defined. The description of the environment must be detailed and should include not only the positive factors of the environment—that is, well-lighted floor space and accessibility of equipment—but also the areas of concern with the person's physical and mental health. For example, if it is the intensive care unit, mental stress and physical endurance can be sorely taxed. Specify if a great deal of walking, lifting, or standing for long periods are involved. No matter how exceptionally well designed the facility is, do not misrepresent the positive and negative variables.

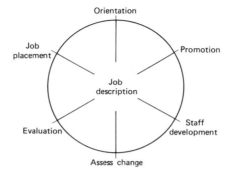

Figure 10-1. Areas for utilization of the job description.

UTILIZATION OF THE JOB DESCRIPTION

The major points to be included in the job description format have been identified and defined. The job description can be used by nursing managers at all levels, in orientation, promotion, staff development, and as a managerial tool to assess change and to evaluate for job placement (1, p. 218) (see Fig. 10-1).

Orientation

The job description can be used as an integral part of the orientation program. It should be properly used by each supervisor to discuss the job description with each new employee so that the duties expected to be performed will be clarified. This can save time and repetition of activities. The job description can be used as a tool for directions if specific clinical areas are designated as orientation areas. For example, one surgical area may be used for orientation of employees who will be assigned to surgical units. This will ease the new employee into the role. Using the job description for orientation in a specific area can also act as a motivating factor for the assigned staff. They will be directly involved with the new employee's orientation, will be familiar with the job description, and may receive personal and professional gratification because of their input in the orientation process.

Promotion

The job description can be fundamental in establishing criteria for promotion within the department.

The job descriptions for all personnel should be available in the clinical setting as a reference for all employees. A staff nurse or nursing assistant, for example, can determine the required qualifications for promotion. The job description allows the employee to set personal goals for growth. The employee knows what is expected in the position she has been hired to fill. In addition, the employee has available, on the assigned unit, job descriptions of positions that may demand more responsibility or specialization. The employee may aspire to one of these positions as she develops her long-range plans. The job description can be a strong incentive for paraprofessionals and nurses who aspire to leadership roles.

Staff Development

The job description can be used to identify the need for position strengthening. For example, if a person has the qualifications for the position but does not meet all the criteria for expected performance, specific intervention might be needed to provide the necessary learning experiences in order to determine if the working potential exists.

Assessment of Change

If the administration wishes to reassign or change the functions and responsibility of staff in a specific area or for the entire department of the organization, the job descriptions would be the selected tools to revamp because of the detailed explanation of positions. For example, in order to create the new position of infection control nurse mentioned earlier in the chapter, an administrative decision had to be made. After the administration made the decision to establish the position, a new job description was developed, and several other already established job descriptions had to be rewritten in order to avoid duplication of activities and to provide for lines of authority and accountability.

Evaluation

If the duties are written clearly and concisely, the reviewer and the employee should be able to determine if the specified criteria have been met. This determination can then be the basis for developing the employee's evaluation, which can be used as a hiring or placement tool.

Job Placement

The required qualifications written in the job description clearly identify the position the applicant is best prepared to handle.

ADMINISTRATIVE ADVANTAGES OF THE JOB DESCRIPTION

Administrators may use the job description to specific advantage.

1. *The job description may be used in a critical review of nursing practice in the clinical setting.* The job description provides administration with the necessary details to identify the strengths and weaknesses of the personnel in a specific area. It provides an opportunity for supervisory personnel to share information with the staff in order to improve patient care.

2. *The job description incorporates standards to maintain continuity of quality care.* The key word is *quality.* Anyone can guarantee that the care will be continued, but the question that arises is "What kind of care?" If the employee is in a supervisory or mangerial capacity, she is accountable not only for her performance but also for the performance of those who are subordinate to her and under her leadership. For example, in team nursing, part of a team leader's responsibility is actively to participate in patient care with her team. In this manner, she is able to determine how the quality of care can be maintained. In addition, the staff (RNs, LPNs, and aides) are charged with the responsibility to report changes in care patterns or the need for revisions of care plans to the team leader. This is clearly stated in the individual job description.

3. *The job description provides a consistent work-flow pattern.* It delineates the responsibilities, functions, and duties of the employee. For

example, if there is any lagging or failing on the part of the employee because she feels she is doing too much, a reference to the job description will clarify the misunderstanding. Everyone employed should be knowledgeable about each specific area of her job description. Dissatisfaction may result if the employee did not take time to read the job description or did not listen and question when it was reviewed before employment.

4. *The job description clearly identifies the communication line.* Who is responsible to whom and what the chain of command is are questions frequently ignored when employees play the game of circumventing lines of authority. When this occurs, there is a breakdown of mutual trust between the employee and the person of line authority. This can be brought to a quick stop if the employee involved is told to review the channel for communication and it is discussed with her. In addition, the person who has been directly affected by the employee's misuse of communication lines must be approached to determine that he is aware of his responsibility to his subordinates.

5. *The job description develops job specifications.* This is a valuable asset for it allows the potential employee and employer to discuss details that have been specifically delineated that may otherwise be overlooked and create a problem for both after the person is employed. The qualifications for the position are clearly spelled out. Either the person meets them or does not.

6. *The job description serves as a basis for staffing.* It can directly affect staffing based on the functions and duties specified in the position the employee holds. There are times when positions are combined and, thereby, some position(s) deleted. Or in other cases, there is the need for a new position and, therefore, an increase in the number of positions. For example, a new intensive care unit is opened. The budgeted staffing is adequate in numbers, but the staff is made up mostly of relatively young RNs. Only the head nurse and her assistant are older and have had several years of experience. Although the young nurses were given a critical care course, this was not enough. It was noted that the nurses were very nervous, edgy, and bickering among themselves about patient care, physicians' orders, patient loads, and so on. Finally, it was suggested that probably what the patients and staff needed was a psychiatric nurse consultant. If it was agreed to implement this suggestion, a job description would be written, and the position added to the staff.

Another instance where staffing is influenced may be the desire to remove all head nurse positions and replace them with clinical specialists who would be responsible for care in several units and with a team leader who would take over many of the head nurse's functions. This change would delete a number of functions and add new ones.

A great deal of time is taken to write a satisfactory job description, and it is not uncommon for the person responsible to use outside sources for suggestions or samples. This consultation may not answer all the employer's needs, but it will provide some insight into writing the job description. It is important mentally to walk through the job yourself. Then draft your walk and have someone who has been in the job critique your data with you. You may find that you walked but you did not see everything along the way. Positions change more frequently than we realize. With the changes being made in health care delivery, we are forced to expand position functions. Many times when we add, we often forget to write it down. That is, we may forget to revise the job description to include the additions.

Too frequently, after job descriptions have been written, we tend to sit back and enjoy the results of a task completed. But after a job description is written, the task has only begun. The writing of a job description is a continuing process. The real challenge is reevaluating and changing the description to accommodate current demands within the nursing care system. Specific times should be set aside to review the descriptions so that one is not faced with an overwhelming task. Plan to review on a scheduled basis, waiting no longer than two years between reviews. Set up a schedule: one month, all RNs; another month, all nursing assistants (depending upon grade); another month, all supervisory positions, and so forth. In this way, job descriptions will no londer be a time-consuming task. The initial work has been accomplished. The bonus is that the employer and employee will know what the expectations are for job performance without referring to "the book."

REFERENCES

1. Swansburg RC: *Management of Patient Care Services*. St. Louis, The CW Mosby Co, 1976, p. 216.
2. Kron T: *The Management of Patient Care,* ed 4. Philadelphia, WB Saunders Co, 1976, p. 25.
3. Public Law 92-603, 92nd Congress, H.R. 1, pp. 101–117, Oct. 30, 1972.

BIBLIOGRAPHY

Periodicals

Driscoll VM: New position description in nursing. *J Nurs Adm* 3:16, November-December 1973.

Donovan HM: Managing the enterprise. *Nurs Service Adm,* St Louis, The CV Mosby Co, 1975.

Francis G: Nursing personnel functions study: who is doing what in the hospital? *Supervisor Nurse* 8:66, April 1977.

Parker JK: Job descriptions of nursing supervisor preamble. *Supervisor Nurse* 9:15, April 1978.

Parker JK: For nursing supervisors. *Supervisor Nurse* 9:37, May 1978.

Tescher BE, Colavecchio R: Definition of a standard for clinical nursing practice. *J Nurs Adm* 7:32, March 1977.

Books

Arndt CH: *Nursing Administration Theory for Practice With a System Approach.* St Louis, The CV Mosby Co, 1975.

Beyers M, Phillips C: *Nursing Management for Patient Care,* ed 2. Boston, Little Brown & Co, 1979.

Kron T: *The Management of Patient Care,* ed 4. Philadelphia, WB Saunders Co, 1976.

11. Staff Evaluation

"Pain or Pleasure"

Mary Ann Miller, R.N.,M.S.N.

BEHAVIORAL OBJECTIVES

After reviewing this chapter, the reader will be able to

- identify the goals of the evaluation process
- utilize the evaluation process to gain useful information for her nursing practice
- utilize the evaluation process to promote self-growth
- describe important elements of evaluation methods
- describe factors that enhance and inhibit the success of the evaluation process

All evaluations of the registered nurses on the staff of this unit must be completed by the end of the month. Please make an appointment to see me. M. Jones, Head Nurse.

All of us have received such notices on countless occasions and should be accustomed to the evaluation process when we are in practice. However, these notices never fail to start our adrenalin flowing and stimulate feelings of dread, resentment, or distaste. Ganong and Ganong (1) present a long list of such frustrations expressed by nurse-managers and employees. Managers refer to inadequate evaluation procedures, unfamiliarity with the person to be evaluated, inadequate time to do evaluations properly, lack of appropriate interviewing and counseling skills. Employees object to the infrequency of evaluation conferences, lack of two-way information sharing with the manager, disregard of their self-development needs, and lack of opportunity to express their opinions about important nursing programs of which they are a part. They are dissatisfied with the lack of performance standards and the use of the same tool to evaluate all levels of personnel.

Generally there is a lack of understanding of the evaluation process —its intent, its necessary components, and methods for ensuring its success. The resulting ineffective use of the process is demonstrated many times by inadequate implementation of inadequate evaluation-tool designs to generate data that are used inappropriately or not at all. The improvement of the evaluation process is an area that requires concerted effort on the part of nurses. All of us are touched by the consequences when it is poorly done.

BACKGROUND INFORMATION

There is a national trend toward quality assurance demanded by the public in all sectors, from "truth-in-lending" laws relative to bank loans to competency-based testing in high schools. Increased awareness and use of legal aid have spotlighted the need for effective evaluation processes in all areas of consumer services. Health care is no exception, and the first step toward its organized evaluation was taken on October 30, 1972, with the passage of Public Law 92-603, which mandated the establishment of PSROs. The JCAH subsequently developed a performance evaluation procedure for use in health care institutions (2).

In the last decade, nurses have been forced to look more seriously at their contributing role in providing health care services. The publication of the American Nurses Association's *Standards for Nursing Practice* and guidelines for their implementation has provided some assurance of consistency in nursing performance within an institution and among similar institutions. It is imperative that nurses continue to set professional standards for nursing because standards are most effective when set by those who practice within that profession and who will be accountable to the set standards for the delivery of quality care. Nonnurses are thus prevented from dictating what quality nursing involves.

NECESSARY FIRST STEPS

It is important to make a distinction between quality assurance (see Chap. 3) and staff evaluation although each relates to the other. The quality assurance program of a health care institution focuses on the overall quality of care provided a client by a variety of individuals. The staff evaluation program examines the quality of an employee's practice in delivering direct or indirect care to a number of clients. In nursing, the staff evaluation program has as its base the stated philosophy of that institution's nursing department and the standards of nursing care derived from that philosophy. These standards are translated into patient care objectives for each nursing unit or division. These objectives provide the road map for meeting the standard of care. Concomitant nursing performance objectives delineate the specific nursing behaviors (activities) required in order to achieve the desired quality of nursing care. For evaluation purposes, these nursing performance standards are the foundation of the performance description against which the employee's performance is judged. The performance description indicates major responsibilities of the nurse to her clients, to her own nurse-manager, to the medical staff, to other department personnel, to committees, to other professional organizations, and to self. It describes those conditions in each area under which performance is satisfactory and thus provides the most obvious criteria for performance evaluation (1, p. 115). Just as patient care objectives (outcomes) are the criteria for evaluating the effectiveness of nursing activity, performance standards are the criteria for evaluating the extent to which the activity is being performed as prescribed (3). The job description is derived from these performance standards and is a more general statement of what the employee is expected to do.

Performance descriptions should be relevant to the role currently expected from the employee (4). In this age of rapid change, performance descriptions should be reviewed at least every two years. They should contain those measurable behaviors that are most important to adequate performance (5). Explicit behavioral terms should be used to identify the expected level of performance — for example, *elicits* relevant history . . . , *documents* in the nursing record . . . , *demonstrates* technical competence in . . . , *explains* to client . . . , *collaborates* with. . . . Many of the items in the performance description will detail the steps of the nursing process in action: assesses, plans, implements, evaluates, modifies.

WHY DO EVALUATIONS?

Staff evaluation is an appraisal of the employee's performance compared with identified criteria (performance standards or performance description). The evaluation can serve a multitude of purposes, far more specific than "letting the staff member know how she is doing." Partridge (6) details them as follows: to provide the employee with recognition for her accomplishments, to discover her professional goals and reconcile them with those of the institution, to improve communication between supervisor and employee and to reach an understanding on job objectives, to determine salary standards and to award merit increases, to select qualified employees for promotion or transfer, to identify unsatisfactory employees for demotion or termination, to determine training and development needs of employees, to establish standards of supervisory job performance, to make inventories of talent within an organization.

It is important that the purpose of the evaluation be clearly communicated to the employee so that she will know how to prepare for the conference and what to expect in the evaluation setting. The purpose determines the focus for the evaluation, influences the choice of method, and indicates the possible responses to the process. For example, there would be differences in the way one would prepare for and conduct or respond to an evaluation for merit salary increases compared to a routine performance evaluation without monetary implications.

WHEN SHOULD EVALUATIONS BE DONE?

Agencies differ in their method of scheduling formal evaluations. Some schedule them on the anniversary of employment. Other agencies schedule evaluations for all staff members in the same month or for certain positions in the same month—for example, all RNs in the month of July, all LPNs in November, all nursing assistants in March. This may be impractical if staff turnover is rapid, since the group being evaluated may include some who have been employed for one year and others only three months. Potential inequities in merit opportunities loom as consequences. When evaluations are spaced adequately, the task for the nurse-manager is not overwhelming in terms of time required to write each one and to meet with each staff member.

Employee performance should be formally evaluated at frequent intervals, initially usually at three months and again at six months. In most cases, evaluation occurs annually thereafter (7). No matter what the schedule is, an employee should feel free to request an evaluation conference whenever necessary. In addition, formal conferences should be scheduled whenever employee performance dictates the need.

Evaluation does not begin when the date for the evaluation conference is set. It begins as soon as the employee accepts a position in the agency. The nurse-manager should immediately acquaint the new employee with the criteria used in the evaluation process. Informal appraisal of the employee's performance should be a continual activity from that point on, with the nurse-manager comparing what she observes to the stated criteria, judging the match, and offering encouragement and constructive suggestions for change to the employee. The nurse-manager should keep a record of these interactions, and one of the best ways she can do this is through the use of the well-documented critical incident or anecdotal note. These notes can be helpful in supplying data to support the formal written evaluation if they meet the following criteria:

- They describe a specific event in behavioral terms.
- They do not contain judgment words.
- They reflect both positive and negative behaviors.
- They identify the persons involved.
- They are dated and signed by both evaluator and employee.

The descriptions contained in anecdotal notes should be concise and complete, including specific statements or dialogue (Fig. 11-1). Such a note will be much more helpful in recalling a situation than a note saying that Mary Jones was rude to a patient or was unwilling to work toward the goals of the unit. If enough notes are written, areas in

---

Name: Mary Jones, Nurse's Aide

Date: 10/5/79

Note: As M. Jones was leaving one of the eight patients assigned to her, Mrs. Brown, a new admission, asked when her doctor would be in and where the bathroom was. M. Jones said, "You are not one of my patients. Put your light on and your nurse will come in."

Joan Smith, Head Nurse 10/5/79

Mary Jones, Nurse's Aide 10/6/79

Figure 11-1.   Anecdotal note

which the employee is performing adequately or inadequately will become obvious. This should provide significant data for the nurse-manager to consider in giving constructive feedback to the employee on a frequent basis. The data should facilitate the job of completing the written evaluation.

WHO DOES THE EVALUATION?

An employee's performance may be evaluated by her peers, her immediate supervisor, or by the employee herself. Peer review is a relatively recent development, becoming more popular with the increasing emphasis on quality assurance and PSROs (7). There have been some problems in developing nursing performance reviews to be used by peers since they require the identification of patient outcomes that are influenced solely by nursing care (2, p. 13). It has been difficult to isolate these factors. Complicating the problem with outcomes assessment in nursing is the focus of nursing care on psychosocial problems that are difficult to measure. In addition, individual professional accountability for the care of specific patients is only slowly becoming a reality with the advent of primary nursing. With the use of the team and functional approaches to delivery of nursing care, it has been difficult to identify an individual nurse as the focus of such a review (8). The case-load approach long used in community health agencies has given those nurses more of an opportunity to use peer evaluations (9).

Evaluation by the nurse-manager is still the most common method and probably will continue to be used as long as nursing care is delivered in ways that place accountability for staff performance and resulting quality of care on those who manage (7). Provisions for employee self-evaluation encourage active participation of the staff member in the evaluation conference. The employee uses the accepted tool to evaluate her own performance prior to the scheduled conference and brings it with her for the purpose of discussing areas of agreement and disagreement, of identifying strengths and weaknesses in her own estimation. MBO encourages the employee to become involved not only in evaluating herself but also in setting her own work goals jointly with her nurse-manager and congruently with stated performance standards (10, 11).

WHICH EMPLOYEE CHARACTERISTICS SHOULD BE INCLUDED?

In the past, most evaluation forms have centered on the personality *traits* of the employee. The judgments about the individual — her initiative, appearance, loyalty, honesty — really relate to her character and can be perceived as a threat to her self-esteem. Since they are not oriented to *events* in which she participates, she can react by becoming self-defensive or by withdrawing from communication (12).

The use of trait characteristics places the evaluator at a disadvantage. Trait language represents the opinion of the evaluator. When the employee disagrees and asks for a specific example, if the evaluator cannot recall a related event, she looks incompetent. Even if the evaluator can identify events, there is no guarantee that both parties will interpret them in the same fashion. Therefore, it is advisable to use event language in the evaluation process, describing specific behaviors rather than personal characteristics (12).

WHICH METHOD SHOULD BE USED?

As Partridge (6, p. 21) points out, there is not a single performance evaluation method that will work well in all settings and with all employees. It depends on the purpose of the evaluation, the work setting, types of personnel, and the kind of work performed. It is crucial to develop a tool that reflects the specific philosophy of the nursing department and relates to the behaviors in the specific performance description. It is not an easy task, but the time will be well spent if the goals of better patient care and satisfied employees are achieved.

The literature on performance appraisal details various methods of evaluation (7, pp. 209–219; 13). Advantages and disadvantages are presented for evaluating staff performance through the use of the essay, graphic rating scale, checklist, critical incident, MBO technique, and work standard. The same treatment is given to those methods used primarily for making decisions about merit increases and promotion: field review, forced-choice rating, ranking, and assessment center. Variations of one or several of these methods may be used in the development of a tool specifically suited to an individual unit or agency.

Regardless of the method chosen or tool developed, some subjective

Table 11-1. Distortions in the Evaluation Process

Halo effect	Observed behavior was positive. Evaluator assumes that all unobserved behavior was just as positive.
Problem distortion or reverse halo effect	One or two negative performances outweigh positive ones. Evaluator is oriented toward negative incidents.
Recency effect	Recent incidents, whether negative or positive, outweigh past performance.
Sunflower effect	Evaluator rates everyone too positively.
Central tendency	Evaluator rates everyone as average. May have insufficient data to do otherwise.
Rater temperament	Different evaluators may be too rigorous or too indulgent.
Guessing error	Evaluator does not actually observe employee but guesses at how she performs.
Contrast error	Evaluator rates employee opposite of how she perceives herself.
Proximity error	Evaluator allows rating on previous item to influence rating on subsequent items.
Hawthorne effect	Employees perform differently when they know they are being evaluated.

Table is adapted with permission from Stevens BJ, *The Nurse as Executive.* Wakefield, Mass, Contemporary Publishing Inc, p. 77, 1975; and from Partridge R, "Evaluating Performance of Nursing Personnel. *Nurs Leadership* 2: 21, September 1979.

judgments creep into the evaluation process and cause distortions in the results. Stevens (5, p. 77) and Partridge (6, p. 21) list ten common errors that evaluators sometimes make (Table 11-1). Partridge (6, p. 22) points out that the number of such errors should decrease as the nurse-manager becomes more comfortable in her role of evaluator and as she develops expertise in handling the evaluation process, whether by additional education or mentor support.

HOW IS THE EVALUATION DONE?

Essential to the effective evaluation is the successful interview, since both evaluator and employee approach it in light of their past evaluation experiences. The interview should be scheduled for a specific time, but that time should be flexible enough so it can be changed, depending on the tempo of the unit. The interview will not be successful if the employee is concerned about completion of her work on time or if she feels she has not fulfilled her responsibilities. An atmosphere of unhurried privacy in a comfortable setting allows both the evaluator and the employee to concentrate on the matter at hand.

The most efficient interview is a two-way process, with each participant being as open as possible to the other's frame of reference, thus encouraging a productive environment. The evaluator and employee should come to the conference well prepared. The evaluator should have in mind a flexible format for the interview. A logical place to begin is with a review of the performance description and of the employee's professional goals. Both individuals can identify the indicated desired behaviors and then begin to share their thoughts on the progress that has occurred.

Discussion at first of the positive aspects of the evaluation ensures that they will be heard. If the negative aspects are discussed first, little of the remaining content will make an impression. Usually there is less chance of threatening the staff member if the evaluator moves from positive aspects to areas in which a change of behavior is desired. It is critical to the success of the whole process that the employee does not receive two conflicting messages — for example, indications that all is well in day-to-day interaction with the nurse-manager and then a written evaluation with many negative comments on it. With such an approach, trust between the nurse-manager and the employee will begin to deteriorate. This can be avoided if the nurse-manager makes it a policy to discuss critical incidents *as they occur,* giving the employee an opportunity to change behavior. There should be *no surprises* at the evaluation conference. Employees have the right to expect that the evaluation will be fair and that there will be positive comments as well as constructive criticism.

The nurse-manager should use evidence from anecdotal records to illustrate the way behavior meets or fails to meet the desired performance standard. Ways in which the employee might achieve desired behavior changes should be discussed. By offering to help the employee in that regard, the manager can enhance the trusting relationship between them. It also indicates that the manager believes that the change is possible and intends to follow through with the recommendation.

The nurse-manager may feel secure enough in her own practice to ask if there is anything she does that interferes with the employee's ability to function at optimum level. If the nurse-manager is sincere in her quest for this input, she can use it to promote her own (and perhaps others') professional growth.

The employee can enhance the two-way responsibility in the evaluation process by asking for input from the nurse-manager concerning ways she can improve her performance. If she is oriented toward the career ladder, she will probably want to know what it is she has to do to be considered for promotion. She should approach the evaluation conference with her own self-evaluation and documentation to support her statements.

The nurse-manager should control the interview and end it within an hour by summarizing what has been said and what is to be done next (5, p. 21). This summary can reveal differences in understanding that need to be clarified. Throughout the process, the nurse-manager should be aware of the interaction that has been occurring, using different interviewing techniques as indicated. She should be aware of common interview traps and work to avoid them (Table 11-2).

Table 11-2. Common Interview Traps

An interview that becomes a one-way conversation

Interruptions of employee's thoughts, explanations, questions

Use of trait language rather than event language

Lack of emphasis on real deficiencies and problems

Expression of opinion before investigation of the facts

Passage of blame for corrective measures to higher authority

Interview that falls into charge-countercharge cycles

Interview that falls into charge-excuse cycles

Interview that deteriorates into social visit

Table is adapted with permission from Stevens BJ, *The Nurse as Executive.* Wakefield, Mass, Contemporary Publishing Inc, 1975, p. 81.

WHAT HAPPENS NEXT?

The evaluation form becomes a part of the employee's permanent record. It must be seen by and discussed with the employee. Both she and the nurse-manager (evaluator) must sign it. The timetable and plan for change in the employee's behaviors that have been mutually agreed upon by the employee and evaluator should also be written, signed, and included. The employee's signature becomes a crucial matter if her termination becomes an issue. If is difficult to prove that the staff member was aware of her poor performance if such evaluations are not signed.

An employee who is in disagreement with the evaluation should be encouraged to write a statement to that effect on the evaluation. If there is no space, she should write her comments on another paper and request that they be included with the completed evaluation form in her permanent record. On occasion, there is a disagreement that cannot be resolved. The employee should avoid bypassing her nurse-manager (evaluator) and going to the supervisor. She should ask that a three-way interview be held to include both the evaluator and the supervisor. All three should strive to keep all comments as objective as possible, focusing on the specific areas of disagreement and avoiding discussion of the personalities involved.

In summary, very few persons take part in the evaluation process with a complete sense of ease. There are actions that will bring the discomfort to a more satisfactory level. These include having an organized process of staff evaluation that identifies goals and employs a tool that indicates the desired behaviors. If the evaluation is shared in an open atmosphere, both the evaluator and the employee should have increased knowledge about themselves and the goals of the unit on which they work. If this is so, then the ultimate goal of better patient care will have been achieved.

REFERENCES

1. Ganong J, Ganong W: *Nursing Management*. Germantown, Md, Aspen Systems Corp, 1976, pp. 108–109.
2. Nursing professional review. *J Nurs Adm* 6:12, November 1976.
3. Cantor MM: *Achieving Nursing Care Standards: Internal and External.* Nursing Resources Inc, Wakefield, Mass, 1978, p. 22.

4. Stevens WF: *Management and Leadership in Nursing.* New York, McGraw-Hill Book Co, 1978, p. 136.
5. Stevens BJ: *The Nurse as Executive.* Wakefield, Mass, Contemporary Publishing Inc, 1975, p. 76.
6. Partridge R: Evaluating performance of nursing personnel. *Nursing Leadership* 2:18, September 1979.
7. Haar LP: Performance appraisal, *The Nurse Evaluator in Education and Service.* New York, McGraw-Hill Book Co, 1978, p. 207.
8. Gold H, Jackson M, et al: Peer review—a working experiment. *Nurs Outlook* 21:634–636, October 1973.
9. Johnson K, Zimmerman MA: Peer review in a health department. *Am J Nurs* 75:619, April 1975.
10. Golightly C: MBO and performance appraisal. *J Nurs Adm* 9:11–20, September 1979.
11. McGregor D: An uneasy look at performance appraisal. *J Nurs Adm* 5:27–31, September 1975.
12. Stevens BJ: First-line patient care management. Wakefield, Mass, Contemporary Publishing Inc., 1976, p. 156.
13. Haar LP, Hicks JR: Performance appraisal: derivation of effective assessment tools. *J Nurse Adm* 6:22–23, September 1976

BIBLIOGRAPHY

Periodicals

Bernhardt J, Schuette L: P.E.T.—a method of evaluating professional nurse performance. *J Nurs Adm* 5:18–21, October 1975.
Brief A: Developing a usable performance appraisal system. *J Nurs Adm* 9:7–10, October 1979.
Corn, F, Magill K: The nursing care audit—a tool for peer review. *Supervisor Nurse* 5:20, February 1974.
Dau G: The appraisal process. *Supervisor Nurse* 7:39, Aguust 1976.
Engle J, Barkauskas V: The evolution of a public health nursing performance evaluation tool. *J Nurs Adm* 9:8–16, April 1979.
Ethridge P, Packard R: An innovative approach to measurement of quality through utilization of nursing care plans. *J Nurs Adm* 6:25, January 1976.
Kabot LB: Objective evaluation for clinical performance. *Supervisor Nurse* 8:16, November 1977.
Kelly RL: Evaluation is more than measurement. *Am J Nurs* 73:114–116, January 1973.
Kopelke CE: The nominal group approach as an evaluation tool. *J Nurs Adm* 6:32, December 1976.
Marriner A: Evaluation of personnel. *Supervisor Nurse* 7:36, May 1976.

Moore TF: Evaluation as a two way street. *Supervisor Nurse* 7:58, June 1976.

Nicholls ME: Quality control in patient care. *Am J Nurs* 74:456–459, March 1974.

Ramey IG: Setting nursing standards and evaluating care. *J Nurs Adm* 3:27, May-June 1973.

Ramphal M: Peer review. *Am J Nurs* 74:63–67, January 1974.

Reider GA: Performance review—a mixed bag. *J Nurs Adm* 4:20–24, May-June 1974.

Stevens BJ: Performance appraisal: what the nurse executive expects from it. *J Nurs Adm* 6:26–31, October 1976.

Watson A, Mayers M: Evaluating the quality of patient care through retrospective chart review. *J Nurs Adm* 6:17, March-April 1976.

Books

Arndt C, Huckabay L: *Nursing Administration—Theory for Practice with a Systems Approach.* St Louis, The CV Mosby Co, 1975.

Clark CC, Shea CA: *Management in Nursing.* New York, McGraw-Hill Book Co, 1979.

Douglas L., Bevis E: *Nursing Leadership in Action.* St Louis, The CV Mosby Co, 1974.

Fivars G, Gosnell D: *Nursing Evaluation: The Problem and the Process.* New York, Macmillan Inc, 1966.

Mager R, Pipe P: *Analyzing Performance Problems.* Belmont, Calif, Fearon-Pitman Publishers Inc, 1970.

Rezler A, Stevens B: *The Nurse Evaluator in Education and Service.* New York, McGraw-Hill Book Co, 1978.

Schneider HL: *Evaluation of Nursing Competence.* Boston, Little Brown and Co, 1979.

12. Fiscal Planning

"To Have or Have Not"

Anthony J. Spinato, F.H.F.M.A.

BEHAVIORAL OBJECTIVES

After reviewing this chapter, the reader will be able to

- list the benefits of a well-coordinated and well-executed budget program
- participate in the construction of operating and capital budgets
- identify how patient care is affected by the budget
- understand why the human element is of major importance in the budgeting process
- identify budgeting as a viable tool in the hands of the user
- assist other health professionals in the management-decision process by analyzing and evaluating variances from budget

Historically, health care agencies have adhered to the adage that "we'll know where we're going when we get there." Structure and organizational planning have not been the order of the day. Survival has more often been dependent upon the philanthropy and humanitarianism of both the community at large and the employees within the health care agency. This philosophy of existence persisted in various forms until the mid-1960s. Then major changes occurred in societal and governmental actions that made it impossible ever again to separate patient care from fiscal responsibility.

RECENT CHANGES IN THE HEALTH CARE AGENCY

Some of the changes that forced this transition were governmental legislation, judicial decisions, advanced technology, and availability of resources.

Perhaps the most significant piece of legislation affecting the health care industry in the United States was the enactment of the Medicare Act of 1965. With the passage of that legislation, the federal government took its first giant step as the designated overseer of this nation's health care delivery system. Authors of the Medicare program significantly underestimated the immediate demand made upon health care agencies and the far-reaching financial burden that the federal government had undertaken.

Within the realm of governmental legislation was the inclusion of health care agencies under the Fair Labor Standards Act, which required agencies to pay minimum wages as well as prescribed overtime rates to employees. Subsequent substantial increases in the minimum wage have had, and will continue to have, significant impact on health care agencies.

Amendments to the Taft-Hartley Act placed health care agencies under the provisions of the NLRA, thereby giving impetus to efforts to unionize health care agencies. More than 60% of total health care agency costs are in the form of salaries and related fringe benefits, whereas salaries and related fringe benefits for industrial enterprises absorb a considerably lower percentage of the budget, somewhere in the area of 25%. Health care agencies, consequently, are very labor intensive.

Within the past five years, landmark judicial decisions have centered around the rights of all people to the best possible medical care, and the right to seek legal recourse when a person feels that the best care has not been provided. Countless millions of dollars have been awarded as a result of malpractice claims. Consequently, the cost of medical profession liability insurance has soared upward of 700% within the past five years. Because of this increase, members of the medical profession find themselves forced to practice defensive medicine by ordering many tests and procedures that normally would not be performed.

Advanced technology that provides new diagnostic and therapeutic equipment, new methods and procedures of treatment, and new career choices have added significantly to mushrooming health care costs.

CAT scanners, which take three-dimensional pictures of the body very quickly, have long been the center of a dispute in the health care field. It is not uncommon for a single CAT scanner to cost more than $600,000. In addition to the capital requirements there is need for additional personnel, which become woven into the fabric of the health care agency.

The "miracles" of modern-day science are not an unmixed blessing. In many areas the effect has been like Pandora's box, releasing new social, ethical and, perhaps above all, financial problems.

All of the factors that have been discussed have played a role in molding the current conditions and attitudes in the health care delivery system as it exists today.

Rising costs have caused public disdain and outcry. The federal government's reaction to this outcry has been reprisal in the form of regulatory controls that have been proclaimed the panaceas of all of the illnesses afflicting the health care delivery system today. The most recent form of such legislation was the proposed hospital cost containment act of 1979 (S.570), which was introduced in Congress in March 1979. That bill represents the administration's approach to the fight against inflation in the hospital sector of our economy. The proposed legislation would establish *voluntary* limits on the annual increases in total hospital expenses and would require *mandatory* limits on the annual increases in hospital inpatient revenues to the extent that the voluntary limits are not effective.

THE NEW PATIENT OF THE EIGHTIES

Perhaps the most critically ill patient today is, in general, the health care delivery system and, in particular, the specific health care agency. Today's health care agency shows symptoms of constipation (inability to eliminate financial waste), fever (rising costs), abdominal pain (federal binding through regulation), and lethargy (employee apathy). If these symptoms are left unchecked, the prognosis for survival is poor. The recommended course of treatment is the establishment, implementation, and maintenance of a responsible system of reporting through planning and budgeting processes, with clear lines of accountability and responsibility. At the heart of budgetary control are the accountability and responsibility of management personnel for each aspect of the operation.

Generally speaking, many people involved in first-level manage-

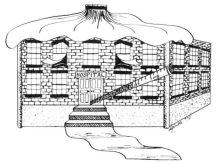

The new "patient" of the eighties.

ment positions, including head nurses and nursing supervisors, have failed to perceive the interrelationships between patient care and cost of care. In fact, there are many misconceptions on the part of this "grass roots" level of management.

The most common misconceptions include the following:

1. The health care agency is making a profit; therefore, all costs can be absorbed by the agency.
2. My *sole* function is the physical and mental well being of the patient. If, through compassion and empathy for the patient, I dispense supplies without charging, no one is hurt.
3. Abuse of sick-leave policy, idleness, and mismanagement of time is a right and does not cost the patient anything.
4. Health care costs are too high, and the patient is being exploited.
5. It doesn't matter how much the agency charges because Blue Cross and Medicare pay for everything. It does not cost anything if Blue Cross or the government pays charges.

The foregoing misconceptions reveal that grass-roots management tends to feel that its actions are insignificant in determining the ultimate quality of care and the fulfillment of the goals of the health care agency. Availability of adequate funds for patient care does not necessarily ensure good patient care. However, the proper distribution of available resources within the health care agency in providing optimum care should be a major objective. No one is in a better position than grass-roots management to assist in providing relevant input data in the budgeting process. This level of management, then, must also be accountable.

The individual qualities and the participation in group action required for management effectiveness must be the same as those qualities and group actions employed in the rendering of effective patient

Table 12-1. The Human Element

	Individual Qualities	Group Action	Product
Patient	Concern	Cooperation	Quality patient care
	Attitude	Organization	
	Resourcefulness	Structure	
	Empathy	Team	
Health Care Agency	Concern	Cooperation	Continued availability of quality patient care
	Attitude	Organization	
	Resourcefulness	Structure	
	Empathy	Team	

care. This interrelationship provides for the optimal availability and usage of patient care resources for, as cost caring decreases, so will the availability of patient care (Table 12-1).

THE BUDGETING PROCESS

Before becoming an active participant in the budgeting program, one must first gain an understanding of the interrelationships involved in the planning activities by the various management levels of the specific health care agency.

The board of trustees has the overall responsibility for the health care agency; consequently, the board, together with top-level management, establishes goals to be followed by the medical staff and the administration. These goals include, but are not limited to, the introduction of new or improved services, long-range capital (building) plans, and outreach services to be provided by the health care agency. The board, then, is the body that determines the role that the agency will play but not necessarily how it will be played.

The administrator, controller, and usually a committee of the medical staff, review the diagnostic and therapeutic services provided by the health care agency within the past few years, and from this data base they attempt to project future patient activity and services based on economic and population changes within the primary service area. Other factors affecting the outcome include services provided by other health care agencies within the same primary service area and the composition of the medical staff.

Assumptions concerning future events and circumstances are reviewed for reasonableness by the board of trustees. After this approval by the board of trustees, the controller (budget director) submits to each department the approved statement of assumptions (i.e., anticipated general activity) for the budget year, together with historical data and statistical information.

Departmental sections (nursing stations) within each department are responsible for the development and intensity of services. These standards of care can be translated into time requirements that will provide anticipated activity for the budget year. The head nurse, with the assistance of nursing supervisors and the director of nursing, completes the budget for the coming year.

Although the accumulation of all budget data into a total facility budget is the responsibility of the controller (budget director), the lowest supervisory level (the head nurse) has as its prime responsibilities the coordinating, communicating, and integrating of all activities that contribute to the accomplishment of the goal. This includes comparing actual results to the budget as well as analyzing deviations from the budget and recommending corrective action when needed.

OBJECTIVES OF BUDGETING

The budgeting process should provide for (1) plans of anticipated activity, (2) a mechanism for measurement of work effort on a timely basis, (3) accountability by someone for variances from budget, and (4) an awareness of costs by all participants in the budgeting program.

THE MAJOR BUDGETS

The budget program contains two major budgets: (1) the operating budget, and (2) the plant and equipment (capital) budget.

The operating budget consists of (*1*) estimates of operating expenses, (*2*) estimates of operating revenues, and (*3*) estimates of activity, expressed in statistical terms or work units.

The plant and equipment (capital) budget consists of estimates of expenditures for (*1*) adding, (*2*) replacing, or (*3*) improving buildings or equipment for the budget period.

THE BUDGET PERIOD

Most health care agencies budget on a monthly basis for a 1-year period. The budget year often begins July 1 and ends June 30, although other 12-month fiscal years are acceptable. Budgeting annually without the ability to compare results monthly does not lend itself to comparisons of actual activity to budget on a timely basis.

Presuming that there is a clear understanding of the value of budgeting, the reader should now be ready to begin participating in the budgeting program. Before doing so, however, it is necessary to have an understanding of cost behavior.

COST BEHAVIOR

All costs fall into three categories: (*1*) fixed, (*2*) semivariable, and (*3*) variable. The categorization of costs depends upon the relationship of cost to volume of activity.

Where there is no relationship of a cost to the volume of activity, the cost is termed *fixed*. A fire insurance premium on a hospital building is an example of a fixed cost. The insurance premium remains constant regardless of the number or types of patients treated in a given period.

A *semivariable* cost has some relationship to volume. For example, three cooks might be required for a patient load of 200 patients per day. However, the addition of 30 patients per day might require an additonal cook.

Variable costs tend to have a direct relationship to volume. An example of a variable cost is food. For each meal served, the total cost of food increases even though total cost per meal might decrease (Fig. 12-1).

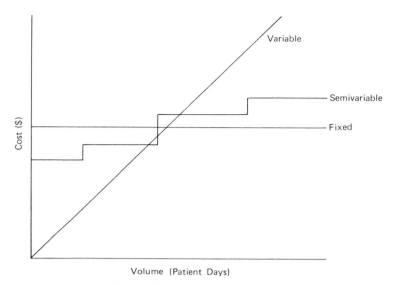

Figure 12-1. Cost behavior.

BUDGET PREPARATION

To explain and review the details of the budgeting and reporting processes, the remaining portion of this chapter will deal with a hypothetical nursing station called Second West. This nursing station contains 30 medical-surgical, adult, acute care beds. Before scheduling of personnel can be determined, it is necessary to obtain from the controller (budget director) an estimate of patient usage of, or activity at, this station. This estimate can be referred to more accurately as the projected work load or volume of this nursing station. The accuracy of the estimate of the projected work load is critical in that the manpower budget is predicated upon work-load requirements.

Assume that 10,215 patient days (the unit of measure denoting lodging facilities provided and services rendered to an inpatient between the census-taking hour on 2 successive days) are to be budgeted for the year. These 10,215 patient days divided by 365 days per year show the average to be 28 patients per day. For a summary of this budget of patient days on a monthly basis, see Table 12-2.

A review of Table 12-2 also reveals that average daily census, on a monthly basis, should range from a low of 22.6 patients per day in August to a projected high of 29.8 patients per day in January through

Table 12-2.   Second West Budget of Patient Days, by Month
For the Fiscal Year July 1, 19____—June 30, 19____

Month	Bed Days Available(A)	Budget of Patient Days(B)	Average Census per Day(C)	Average % of Occupancy(D) (B÷A)
July	930	850	27.4	91.4
August	930	700	22.6	75.3
September	900	860	28.7	95.6
October	930	905	29.2	97.3
November	900	800	26.7	88.9
December	930	840	27.1	90.3
January	930	925	29.8	99.5
February	840	835	29.8	99.4
March	930	925	29.8	99.5
April	900	875	29.2	97.2
May	930	900	29.0	96.8
June	900	800	26.7	88.9
Total	10,950	10,215	28.0	93.3%

(A) Bed days available equal number of days in each month times 30 beds available per day.
(B) From controller (budget director).
(C) Budget of patient days per month divided by number of calender days per month.
(D) Average census per day divided by 30 beds/day or (B) divided by (A).

March. There is no indication of the anticipated census for any "typical" day, should one exist, since average daily census on a monthly basis does not give any consideration to specific high-low daily activity. Nursing standards for staffing will be predicated on average daily patient utilization.

Assume that nursing standards for staffing at various average patient levels have been developed for this nursing station (see Table 12-3). Standards for staffing range from a low of 17 patients per day to a high of 30 patients per day. A review of Table 12-3 will reveal the incremental requirements of nursing personnel at each patient level within the relevant range. Semivariable nursing costs are thus evidenced. The standards, in this instance, were developed by the head nurse and nursing supervisor, and were approved by the director of nursing service.

The main concern at this point is the conversion of patient volume into manpower resource requirements. It now becomes evident that any attempt to convert projected patient days into manpower resource

Table 12-3. Second West Nursing Standards for Staffing at Various Average Daily Patient Levels For the Fiscal Year July 1, 19—June 30, 19—

Average Number of Patients per Day	Total Hours per Pay Period	Ratio of Paid Hours per Patient Day	Weekdays											Weekends								
			Shift 1 (Days)					Shift 2 (Eves.)			Shift 3 (Nites)			Shift 1			Shift 2			Shift 3		
			HN	RN	LPN	Aide ORD	Unit Sec	RN	LPN	Aide ORD	RN	LPN	Aide ORD	RN	LPN	Aide ORD	RN	LPN	Aide ORD	RN	LPN	Aide ORD
30	1,762	4.20	1	3	3	1	1	1	1	1	1	1	1	2	2	1	1	1	1	1	1	1
29	1,762	4.34	1	3	3	1	1	1	1	1	1	1	1	2	2	1	1	1	1	1	1	1
28	1,671	4.26	1	3	2	1	1	1	1	1	1	1	1	2	2	1	1	1	1	1	1	1
27	1,671	4.26	1	3	2	1	1	1	1	1	1	1	1	2	2	1	1	1	1	1	1	1
26	1,580	4.34	1	2	2	1	1	1	1	1	1	1	1	2	2	1	1	1	1	1	1	1
25	1,453	4.15	1	2	1	1	1	1	1	1	1	1	1	2	1	1	1	1	1	1	1	1
24	1,453	4.32	1	2	1	1	1	1	1	1	1	1	1	2	1	1	1	1	1	1	1	1
23	1,453	4.51	1	2	1	1	1	1	1	1	1	1	1	2	1	1	1	1	1	1	1	1
22	1,326	4.31	1	1	1	1	1	1	1	1	1	1	1	1	1	1	1	1	1	1	1	1
21	1,326	4.51	1	1	1	1	1	1	1	1	1	1	1	1	1	1	1	1	1	1	1	1
20	1,326	4.74	1	1	1	1	1	1	1	1	1	1	1	1	1	1	1	1	1	1	1	1
19	1,326	4.98	1	1	1	1	1	1	1	1	1	1	1	1	1	1	1	1	1	1	1	1
18	1,235	4.90	1	1	1		1	1	1	1	1	1	1	1	1	1	1	1	1	1	1	1
17	1,235	5.19	1	1	1		1	1	1	1	1	1	1	1	1	1	1	1	1	1	1	1

[a] Budget for the fiscal year is based on an average of 28 patients per day.

Table 12-4. Second West (30 Beds) Hours Requirements Budget Occupancy 28 Patients/Day (Normal Staffing) For the Fiscal Year July 1, 19—June 30, 19—

Weekdays	Hours/Year	Weekends	Hours/Year	Total Hours/Year
Days				
Head Nurse	(2,086)			2,086
3 Registered Nurses	(6,258)	2 Registered Nurses	(1,668)	7,926
2 Licensed Practical Nurses	(4,172)	2 Licensed Practical Nurses	(1,668)	5,840
1 Aide/Orderly	(2,086)	1 Aide/Orderly	(834)	2,920
1 Unit Secretary	(2,086)		–	2,086
Total – Days	(16,688)		(4,170)	20,858
Evenings				
1 Registered Nurse	(2,086)	1 Registered Nurse	(834)	2,920
1 Licensed Practical Nurse	(2,086)	1 Licensed Practical Nurse	(834)	2,920
1 Aide/orderly	(2,086)	1 Aide/Orderly	(834)	2,920
Total – Evenings	(6,258)		(2,502)	8,760
Nights				
1 Registered Nurse	(2,086)	1 Registered Nurse	(834)	2,920
1 Licensed Practical nurse	(2,086)	1 Aide/Orderly	(834)	2,920
1 Aide/Orderly	(2,086)	1 Aide/Orderly	(834)	2,920
Total – Nights	(6,258)		(2,502)	8,760
Grand Total Hours Required	(29,204)		(9,174)	38,378
Sick, Vacation, Holiday, From Pool (13.5% × 38,378) (See Table 12-5)				5,181
Total Hours Charged to Unit (Hours Paid)				45,559
Patient Days				10,215
Hours Paid Per Patient Day = 43,559 ÷ 10,215				4.26

requirements is, at best, a most difficult assignment. Various alternatives are possible:

1. *Prepare the budget on the assumption of monthly staffing requirements.* In other words, July will require a staff based on 28 patients per day. In August, the staff requirements will be based on 23 patients per day. If the budget is to be based on average monthly requirements, what is to be done with the additional personnel required in July (1 RN, 1 LPN on day shift during the week, and 1 LPN on day shift on weekends) that probably are not needed during the month of August at this nursing station? It might behoove the head nurse to schedule a significant amount of vacation in August, when the average daily census appears to be the least demanding. It is relevant to note that, even with an average census of 23 patients per day in August, it is possible that some days during that period will exceed 28 patients per day, so the head nurse must be flexible.

2. *Prepare the budget on the assumption of 28 patients per day for each day of the year.* Peaks and valleys are almost certain to exist under this method. There is a likelihood that there will be deviations in actual monthly activity from planned activity, but it will be more likely that the average census for the year will approximate 28 patients per day.

For purposes of this budget, it will be assumed that normal staffing will be based on an average census of 28 patients per day. Given the nursing standard for 28 patients per day (Table 12-3), staffing is converted into hours requirements for the fiscal year (Table 12-4). Note that each full-time employee is paid for an average of 2,086 hours per year, which is roughly 52 weeks per year times 5 workdays per week. After having vacation, sick leave, and holiday time, a full-time employee will work approximately 1,806 hours per year. This means that nursing coverage for nonproductive scheduled time (vacation, sick, and holiday) must come from another area. For our purposes, a nursing pool has been established to provide this coverage for all medical-surgical areas. In this case study, some 5,181 hours will be required of pool personnel to accomplish this task.

Nonproductive paid compensation is often calculated as a percentage of total compensation. In our illustration, it will be 13.5% of total work hours required.

After the projected needs of each nursing station within the medical-surgical areas are determined, a schedule of availability of nursing personnel versus demands that will be placed upon the pool will be prepared (Table 12-5). Note that the 22 positions available in the nursing pool are inadequate to cover vacation, sick, and holiday time for all

Table 12-5. Medical Surgical Areas Nursing Pool Budget
For the Fiscal Year July 1, 19____–June 30, 19____

		Hours
Personnel Available		
(7) Registered Nurses		14,602
(11) Licensed Practical Nurses		22,946
(4) Aides/Orderlies		8,344
Total Hours Paid		45,892
Less: Sick, Vacation, Holiday (13.5%)		(6,195)
Hours Available for Other Areas		39,697
Requirements:		
Medical and Surgical Area	*Hours*	
Second West (To Table 12-4)	5,181	
Second East	6,250	
Third North	8,100	
First South	4,211	
Second South	9,750	
Third South	12,500	
Total Hours Required		45,992
Projected (Shortage)/Overage		(6,295)

medical-surgical areas. The projected shortage of 6,295 hours approximates 3 positions that should be filled before the beginning of the fiscal year. The composition of the 45,992 required total pool hours must be established and evaluated to determine which positions (RNs, LPNs, aid-orderlies) to hire for.

Nursing Station Second West will absorb costs, then, of its own personnel as well as of personnel assigned from the medical-surgical nursing pool. Table 12-4 shows that 43,559 hours will be budgeted for the fiscal year. Since some 10,215 patient days are budgeted, this is the equivalent of 4.26 paid hours per patient day. This number of hours paid per patient day is our first indicator of the reasonableness or unreasonableness of the budget. However, there is no absolute number or standard hours per patient day that should be expended to provide adequate patient care. All that can be relied upon are ranges of acceptability. Medical-surgical indices range from 3 to 6 hours per patient day. This means that the present budget appears to be well within normal limits.

After the hours requirements have been determined, a payroll budget worksheet (Table 12-6) should be completed by the head nurse. This worksheet will provide for all positions budgeted for the coming budget year. The listing will be in job classification sequence, such as

Table 12-6. Second West Payroll Budget Worksheet
For the Fiscal Year July 1, 19____–June 30, 19____

Prepared by: _____   Approved by: _____   Department:_____

Payroll Position Budgeted	Shift	Reg. Hours pp	Annual Hours	Hourly Rate		Other Cost per Hour*	Total Annual Cost	
Head Nurse								
O'Connell, K. B.	D	80	2,086	6	50		13,559	00
Total Head Nurse			2,086	(1)			13,559	00 (1)
Registered Nurses								
Days:								
Baker, C. T.		80	2,086	6	10		12,724	60
Collins, A. M.	D	80	2,086	5	95		12,411	70
Dollen, F. M.	D	40	1,043	5	75		5,997	25
Heartz, D. E.	D	40	1,043	5	70		5,945	10
Open	D	32	834	5	70		4,753	80
Kline, C. L.	D	32	834	5	70		4,753	80
Total Day Shift		304	7,926				46,586	25
Evenings:								
Fox, H. E.	E	80	2,086	5	80	25	12,620	30
Stover, T. E.	E	16	417	5	75	25	2,502	00
Tilly, A. M.	E	16	417	5	70	25	2,502	00
Total Evening Shift		112	2,920				17,624	30
Nights:								
Evans, B. A.	N	80	2,086	5	80	20	12,516	00
Torry, G. D.	N	32	834	5	75	20	4,962	80
Total Night Shift		112	2,920				17,478	30
Total "Core"—Reg. Nurse			13,766	(1)			81,688	85 (1)

Total annual cost equals hourly rate plus other cost per hour times annual hours.
*Shift differential.

(1) To Table 12-7.

RN, LPN. Open positions (approved vacant positions) will be listed in the appropriate category. Depending on the hours requirements schedule, manpower needs might warrant (1) the hiring of or transferring in of personnel; (2) the transfer of current personnel to other areas; (3) the laying off of personnel; (4) the changing of employee status: full time to part time, or part time to full time; or (5) the closing of previously approved open positions. In this case study, there is one open

Table 12-7. Second West Payroll Budget (Hours and Dollars)
For the Fiscal Year July 1, 19_____–June 30, 19_____

	Core		Pool		Payroll Budget Total	
Position	Hours (1)	$ (2)	Hours (3)	$ (4)	Hours (5)	$ (6)
Head Nurse	2,086	$13,559	–	–	2,086	$13,559
Registered Nurse	13,766	81,689	2,086	$12,400	15,852	94,089
Licensed Practical Nurse	11,680	49,900	1,769	7,610	13,449	57,510
Aide & Orderly	8,760	32,000	1,326	4,900	10,086	36,900
Unit Secretary	2,086	7,650	–	–	2,086	7,650
Totals	38,378	$184,798	5,181	$24,910	43,559	$209,708

(1) Table of Hours Requirements or Payroll Budget Worksheet – Table 12-4 or Table 12-6.
(2) Payroll Budget Worksheet – Table 12-6.
(3) Table of Hours Requirements and Controller.
(4) Controller.
(5) Column (1) plus (3).
(6) Column (2) plus (4).

part-time RN position that should be filled to meet the hours requirements.

The hourly rate of pay is obtained from the controller (budget director). The rate of pay should be representative of the average rate at which the employee will be paid in the budget year. This might include a cost of living and/or merit increase.

Total core hours and core dollars are transferred to the payroll budget of hours and dollars (Table 12-7).

The budget for fringe benefits (including FICA, health insurance, life insurance, pension benefits, etc.) is generally furnished by the controller (budget director). Fringe benefits are for the most part a function of salaries and wages.

Medical and surgical supplies and other supplies are often budgeted on a cost per patient day. Patient mix contributes significantly to the use of supplies. Again, the controller (budget director) plays a role in developing these budget items.

The operating budget for Second West is presented in Table 12-8. Estimates of operating revenue are not shown as a part of this budget. Generally, the estimates of revenue are a responsibility of the controller (budget director). The estimate of revenue will, of course, be based on the estimate of patient days budgeted for the fiscal year (10,215 times the rate per patient day). The rate, often referred to as the room rate, will be set high enough to absorb the direct cost per patient day of the department ($25.40) plus costs including, but not limited to, dietary patient meals, laundry, housekeeping, medical records, utilities, depreciation on building, administration, and admissions. Accountability for these component costs will, of course, be the responsibility of other sections and departments within the health care agency.

It should be evident now that management from each section of the health care agency provides the bricks and mortar upon which the foundation of the budget program is established. It is relevant to mention at this point that the responsibility of the head nurse should be geared more to accountability of hours rather than of dollars. The nurse has little or no input to the salary levels of nursing personnel, the granting of an across-the-board increase, and so forth. The head

Table 12-8. Second West Annual Operating Budget
For the Fiscal Year July 1, 19____–June 30, 19____

Patient Days	10,215	(A)
Hours Paid	43,559	(B)
Direct Costs		
Salaries and Wages	$209,708	(C)
Fringe Benefits	35,389	
Medical-Surgical Supplies	12,000	
Other Supplies	2,400	
Total Direct Costs	$259,497	(D)
Direct Cost per Patient Day	$ 25.40	(E)
Direct Cost per Paid Hour	$ 5.96	(F)

(A) From Table 12-2, Column B.
(B) From Table 12-4 or Table 12-7.
(C) From Table 12-7.
(E) (D) divided by (A).
(F) (D) divided by (B).

nurse, however, must be aware of the cost of running her area because committing hours (over which there is control) is spending dollars. The head nurse should be the best judge of severity of need for nursing on her unit. An imbalance in care and need can prove costly, not purely financially speaking, but certainly with strong adverse medical and financial overtones. The imbalance in care can cause (*1*) treatment delays and complications; (*2*) patient, physician, and employee complaints; (*3*) services needed but not provided; (*4*) a decrease in the quality of nursing care—all of which inevitably will lead to staff absenteeism and turnover.

The annual budget is now complete for Second West (Table 12-8). However, this budget on a responsibility basis is now incorporated as a part of the aggregate medical-surgical budget (Table 12-9), which in turn is a component of the overall nursing service budget.

Table 12-9. Medical Surgical Budget
For the Fiscal Year July 1, 19____–June 30, 19____

	Amount		
Salaries and Wages	$ 28,000		
Fringe Benefits	4,700		
Other Supplies	300		
Total Own Operations	$ 33,000		
Nurses Station			
2 - W	$259,497	(A)	
2 - E	275,200		
2 - S	221,425		
3 - N	197,258		
Total Nurses Stations	$953,380		
Total All Direct Costs	$986,380		

			Nurses Station
	Patient		*Direct Cost per*
Nurses Station	*Days*		*Patient Day*
2 - W	10,215	(B)	$25.40 (C)
2 - E	10,800		25.48
2 - S	8,750		25.31
3 - N	7,900		24.97
Total Patient Days	37,665		$25.31

(A), (B), (C) from Table 12-8.

MONTHLY BUDGET

After the annual operating budget has been completed, the monthly budget should be developed. In developing this budget, it will be assumed that the hours paid for any given month will be determined by dividing the number of days in the month by the number of days in the fiscal year times the annual budgeted hours. For example, there are 31 days in July; then 31 days divided by 365 days per year times 43,559 hours paid per year, which equals 3,700 paid hours for July (Table 12-10). The above example will generally be representative of a normal scheduling pattern by nursing, which is typically prepared on a 6-week rotating basis. Ideally, hours requirements should be related to patient days. If this concept were followed, hours paid in July would be determined by the ratio of July patient days to total patient days times total annual hours, or

$$\frac{850}{10,215} \times 43,559 = 3,625 \text{ hours.}$$

Under this method, every month during the fiscal year will be budgeted at 4.26 hours per patient day. The graph in Figure 12-2 illustrates this point.

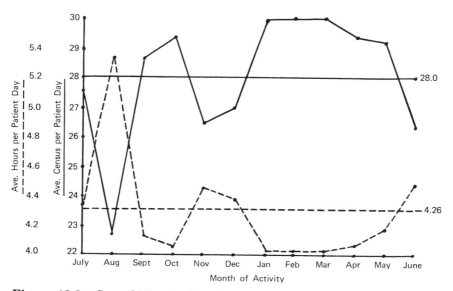

Figure 12 2. Second West budgeted average census per patient day (by month) versus budgeted average hours per patient day (by month).

The summary of budget paid hours per patient day (Table 12-10) is a by-product of the monthly hours paid budget and patient days monthly budgets. Significant monthly variations in paid hours per patient day are evidenced. Ranges are 4.00 paid hours per patient day for the period January through March, which compares favorably to 5.29 paid hours per patient day budgeted in August.

A great number of health care agencies use paid hours per patient day to compare their medical-surgical activity, intensive care activity, and so forth against other health care agencies of comparable size.

Comparisons are also made by health care agencies on the components of the paid hours per patient day. For example, RN hours per patient day might be higher and LPN hours per patient day might be lower than in other agencies, although the aggregate hours might be essentially the same. A difference in composition might be evidenced by comparing paid dollars per patient day.

There is a relationship between hours paid and salaries and wages. Consequently, salaries and wages for July will equal $17,810, calcu-

Table 12-10. Second West Summary of Budget Hours per Patient Day, by Month
For the Fiscal Year July 1, 19____–June 30, 19____

Month	Hours Paid (A)	Patient Days (B)	Paid Hours per Patient Day (C)
July	3,700	850	4.35
August	3,700	700	5.29
September	3,580	860	4.16
October	3,700	905	4.09
November	3,580	800	4.48
December	3,700	840	4.40
January	3,700	925	4.00
February	3,339	835	4.00
March	3,700	925	4.00
April	3,580	875	4.09
May	3,700	900	4.11
June	3,580	800	4.48
Total	43,559	10,215	4.26

(A) Days in month divided by days in fiscal year multiplied by 43,559 hours paid.
(B) From Table 12-2.
(C) (A) divided by (B).

lated as follows: July hours divided by total annual hours times annual salaries and wages, or 3,700 divided by 43,559 times $209,708. Fringe benefit costs are often allocated on the same basis as salaries and wages.

Medical, surgical, and miscellaneous supplies bear a relationship to the number of patients and the type of patient. For this illustration, the annual budget for these costs will be divided equally into each month of the fiscal year.

It is necessary that the reader understand that the budget is the product of the nursing station and that actual results will be compared to budget on a monthly basis. It was stressed that accountability is an essential ingredient in any viable management system. Explanation of variances from the budget are to be given by the head nurse.

EXPLANATION OF VARIANCES

Each month, as actual data become available, the head nurse will be furnished with a comparative performance report, which compares the actual results with what was budgeted. The report will be similar to that presented in Table 12-11. To assist the head nurse in evaluating performance, supportive detail reports of actual costs will be provided. These reports will generally summarize all personnel hours, by employee, charged to the nursing station. Vacation, sick leave, and holiday hours, as well as salary dollars, should also be furnished.

A review of the comparative performance report for the month of July (Table 12-11) illustrates that there were 50 patient days less than budgeted. At the same time,   Second West was charged for 50 hours more than were budgeted.

Salaries and wages and fringe benefits exceeded budget, whereas supplies expenses were under budget for the month.

Does a review of the above information necessarily indicate that an unfavorable performance existed? It is not possible to respond accurately to this question without first reviewing actual cost data, which will provide the basis for answers to other questions, such as the following: How many hours were worked during the month? How many hours and dollars of nonproductive time (sick leave, vacation, and holiday) were charged to Second West during the month of July? Does paid nonproductive time exceed the percentage budgeted? If so, is the variance in the form of extended sick leave, or for vacation, being taken in excess of the budget? Was any nonproductive time taken for which the nursing pool was not called on to cover?

Table12-11. Second West Comparative Performance Report, Budget
Versus Actual
For the Month of July 19____

	Budget	Actual	Under/ Over Budget
Patient Days	850	800	50
Hours Paid	3,700	3,750	(50)
Salaries and Wages	$17,810	$18,100	$(290)
Fringe Benefits	2,982	3,040	(58)
Medical-Surgical Supplies	1,000	945	55
Other Supplies	200	190	10
Total Direct Costs	$21,992	$22,275	$(283)
Direct Cost per Patient Day (A)	$ 25.87	$ 27.84	$(1.97)
Direct Cost per Hour (B)	$ 5.94	$ 5.94	$ -

Explanation of variations from budget to be completed by head nurse:
(A) Total direct costs divided by patient days (21,992 ÷ 850); (22,275 ÷ 800).
(B) Total direct costs divided by hours paid (21,992 ÷ 3,700); (22,275 ÷ 3750).

A review of cost data from the payroll department might well reveal that vacation taken during the month of July was more than had been budgeted, since vacation was budgeted as being taken evenly throughout the fiscal year. This being the case, actual costs in future months should fall below budget (all other things being equal).

THE CAPITAL BUDGET

Under normal circumstances, health care agencies exist in an environment typified by resource scarcity for the acquisition of capital equipment. Much of the technical equipment used by the health care agency does not lend itself to mass production. It is not uncommon to expend funds of $60,000 to $100,000 or more for individual pieces of diagnostic equipment used in the departments of pathology and radiology. Inflation has played a significant role in causing cost increases of equipment. A great deal of equipment becomes obsolete quickly due to continued advances in technology.

Budget Year _____   Department _____

Type and Description of Equipment Requested: Priority — Circle
                                                                   One
                                                              1. Urgent
                                                              2. Essential
                                                              3. Economically
                                                                 Desirable
                                                              4. Generally
                                                                 Desirable

---

Number   Unit Cost   Estimated Cost   Check Appropriate Block:
of Units

                                            Addition ☐   Replacement ☐

Item To Be Replaced:
          Make: Model: Age: Approximate Value:

Will purchase of this equipment create additional expense in another part of
your budget?

                          Yes _ _ _   No _ _ _

Explain: Approximate Yearly Cost $:

Figure 12-3.   Capital expenditure request.

Typically, there are more requests for equipment than funds available to satisfy needs of the health care agency. It is an everyday occurrence for requests for equipment to exceed available funds by a five
to one ratio. Since this condition is often a way of life, the health care
agency, through its long-range planning committee, must act with
good judgment in attempting to evaluate capital requests. Requests
can best be evaluated on a priority basis. The priorities could very well
be (1) urgent, (2) essential, (3) economically desirable, and (4) generally desirable. Priorities are established by each department based
upon its function.

   In the department of nursing, for example, the priority given to a
piece of equipment by the head nurse could vary significantly from the

Period: July 1, 19___ June 30, 19___

Department: _____

Item No: (1)	Description of Item	A/R (2)	Quantity	Date Req'd.	Estimated Cost

(1) List in order of priority.
(2) A = Addition, R = Replacement.

Figure 12-4. Proposed capital expenditure budget.

priority ultimately assigned by the director of nursing. The head nurse should initially assign priorities for her particular nursing station. A capital expenditure request form (Fig. 12-3) will be completed for each capital item requested. Unit costs are generally obtained from the purchasing director. Information relating to the capital item to be replaced, if applicable, is obtained from the controller's office.

The proposed capital expenditure budget (Fig. 12-4) from the nursing department represents the summation of capital expenditure requests (Fig. 12-3) originating from each nursing area.

The provision of substantial resources for the development and implementation of a sophisticated budget program that does not also provide for that all-important ingredient, the human element, is almost certainly destined for failure. Attaining a basic understanding of the budgeting process and its acceptance by grass-roots managers is of paramount importance if any success is to be achieved.

The budgeting process is merely a tool in the hands of people. But, like any other tool, its efficient use depends upon training, practice, skill and, perhaps above all, acceptance and understanding.

BIBLIOGRAPHY

Berman HJ, Weeks LE: *The Financial Management of Hospitals,* ed 3, Ann Arbor, Health Administration Press, 1976, Chap. 15.

Budgeting Procedures for Hospitals. Chicago, American Hospital Association, 1971, Chaps. 2, 5, and 7.

Seawell LV: *Hospital Financial Accounting Theory and Practice.* Chicatgo, Hospital Financial Management Association, 1975, Chap. 6.

13. Labor-Management Relations in Health Care Delivery

"A Basic Understanding"

Joyce L. Schweiger, R.N., M.S.

BEHAVIORAL OBJECTIVES

Upon reviewing this chapter, the reader will be able to

- list five factors of labor relations philosophy that could be incorporated to facilitate a workable labor-management relationship
- identify the nine areas the nurse-manager should be knowledgeable about in the unionization process
- list five factors that predispose a nursing staff toward unionization
- compare the attitudes of administrators and nursing directors toward unionization (collective bargaining)
- identify the indirect effect unionization can have in delivery of quality patient care

Involvement with unions and unionization for many years has been an issue that management in the health care field has often tried to ignore, to avoid, and intentionally to bypass. With the growing concern for quality care, patients' rights, workers' rights, plus the increase in bureaucratic expansion in the health care industry, unions and unionization have become a very real issue.

In 1974, then-President Richard M. Nixon signed Public Law 93-360, the amendment to the National Labor Relations Act (NLRA). For the first time, all nongovernmental health care agencies were placed under the same umbrella by federal labor laws (1). The addition of Public Law 93-360 to the NLRA presented immediate and significant concerns to all health care agencies.

One concern was a projected increase in unionization activities; another was that administrators of health care agencies were required to operate under "a complex body of statutory, administrative and case law" (1, pp. 1–2).

Under these circumstances, it has now become impossible to separate the topic and issues of labor from personal administration and labor relations. As a result, managers in health care institutions have had to become familiar with the functions and structure of the NLRA. In doing this, a new philosophy has to be devised and implemented — one that will be less biased and more realistic in its concept of labor relations (unionization). This alteration in thought is a time-consuming task, not to be taken lightly by either of the parties.

Strong negative feelings have existed and grown over the years in regard to management's acceptance of unions and unionizations. This feeling has existed as part of their organizational framework, but the negativism is not only on the part of management but also within labor unions.

ATTITUDE OF MANAGEMENT TOWARD UNIONS

In 1978, Sargis (2) described a study that was undertaken to determine the feelings of directors of nursing toward professional associations, professional authority, and collective bargaining. The participants were limited to directors in nonprofit hospitals in New York, New Jersey, and Connecticut (primary nonorganized sectors of the hospital industry). A total of 397 directors were involved. A mail-back questionnaire survey was used. Areas of the data collected indicated that, although the directors chose a middle-of-the road attitude toward the professional association as a collective bargaining agent and accepted the concept of professional authority in the decision-making process, they did not all entirely accept the process of collective bargaining. In general, the directors were unsympathetic to the total concept of collective bargaining. This implies that nursing directors, as Sargis (2, p. 26) says, "will not be a central force in future collective bargaining by registered nurses in this country."

Findings in another study conducted and reported in 1978 by Samaras (3) lead one to believe conclusively that management must take a long, hard, objective look at its attitude toward labor unions and consider ways to cope with them. In this study, which was limited to the administrators of three southwestern medical centers, the data collected were based upon replies to ten open-ended questions related to unionization. At the conclusion of the study, the findings indicated that the administrators felt that unions were a restraint on management, that they increased costs and looked for shortcomings within management to scrutinize. Despite this general tendency toward a negative outlook, the administrators did not suggest that unions and unionization would decrease but rather implied that they would increase in the future.

Two interesting observations related to both study findings are, first that the attitude of both representatives of management — directors of nursing and administrators — tended to be negative in relation to collective bargaining and, second that they too will not expedite collective bargaining in hospitals.

FIVE FACTORS OF LABOR RELATIONS PHILOSOPHY

On the other hand, the attitude of labor toward management has been, in most cases, suspicious and negative. Labor union representatives who have been requested to interview in a facility have taken little time to investigate thoroughly the reasons behind the request for possible unionization. Usually an all-out effort is made to increase the wedge between management and staff. Also, depending upon the size of the health care agency, if one sector is inclined toward unionization, the union representatives will encourage the interested pro-union worker to infiltrate into other sectors that are uninvolved, so the movement will gain strength and momentum. This is expected behavior. Many of the tactics used by labor representatives, in an attempt to unionize an agency or a sector of one, are carried over to the bargaining table between labor and management. In many situations, these tactics will set the tempo for a continued relationship of antagonism between union and management. A situation that could probably be alleviated is at least eased if a change in attitude is encouraged by both parties.

One of the primary steps to take in order to facilitate a change in the attitudes of management and labor would be to establish an air of objectivity in their mutual thought processes. The tendency in the past has been one of perpetuating antagonism through emotional responses when the two factions have met.

In 1977, Werther and Lockhart (4) presented five factors that are considered a part of labor relations philosophy:

1. The survival of the employee is the paramount goal.
2. Administration at all levels must recognize the survival needs of the employee association, its leaders and members.
3. Workers, professionals, and their leaders must respect the employees' need for efficiency and effectiveness.
4. Problem solving should be undertaken jointly with a pragmatic, not an ideological outlook.
5. Cooperation is the most viable long-term strategy for all parties.

The interpretation of these five factors may vary from situation to situation or between union and health care agencies, but should be taken into account by management in developing its philosophy of labor relations.

Survival of the Employee

Survival of the employee cannot be stated in more definitive terms. It can be interpreted in two ways. If the health care agency has excessive duress placed upon it by the demanding parties, it can be forced to become nonexistent. The demands will outweigh the supply (cost, available staff, space, etc.) and, as a result, there will be no need for employees or employee representation. However, if the employee is very negative, unwilling to listen, and has made prejudgments in relation to demands, those workers requesting the hearing can take another step—they can strike. A strike would cause havoc for the health care agency and ultimately affect the employee, particularly over a long period.

Administration's Recognition of Survival Needs

When management makes a decision that will directly affect the worker, management must consider whether this will change the worker's standard of living and work load, and affect his self-image. It is essential for management to consider the basic needs of people, the first of which is survival.

Need for Efficiency and Effectiveness

The employee's feelings of self-esteem and self-image must be a prime consideration by all parties when any decisions are made. The worker must feel a part of the decision-making process and be willing to be accountable for her part in the outcome of mutual decisions.

Problem Solving (Unity in Decisions)

As mentioned in Chapter 6, problem solving should not be a one-person process or a one-faction process. This process is even more emphatically stressed when there is a union or other professional organization involved within the health care agency. The seven-step problem-solving process may take longer because of the number of persons involved but, in the end, the results will be more satisfying and the solutions more acceptable to both parties if there is equal representation.

Cooperation between Labor and Management

Cooperation has always been a key factor in any type of relationship. Therefore, it should be a primary concern to both labor and management. A lack of cooperation is particularly crucial to the health care industry because lack of cooperation results in failure to perform at acceptable levels and the patient suffers. The existing social structure today fosters the concept of cooperation through free expression of thought on many and varied levels. The health care industry is a part of this structure, as in labor. Each has its own goals, but both supposedly have the same ultimate goal—patients' welfare, which can only be achieved through a cooperative effort. If the free expression of thought were expanded to include listening and hearing on the part of both labor and management, perhaps the final outcome would be objectivity in thought that would lend to a cohesive working relationship.

INDIRECT EFFECT OF UNIONIZATION ON PATIENT CARE

There are expected and unexpected factors that come with unionization. Each of them will have an effect on direct patient care. Two of these factors are workers' job descriptions and the attitude of workers, as union members, toward their jobs.

Job descriptions have been discussed in Chapter 10; however, the importance of the structure and contents of the job description becomes a major issue, particularly in the presence of unionization. Nurses, aides, technicians, and other health workers must be knowledgeable about the specific functions and duties of the position they are assigned to. The employer or his designated representative must be certain that the job description is detailed enough to avoid gaps and overlap in functions and duties that may be considered or labeled at a later time as unfair and unjust practice. The wise administrator will not hesitate, if there is a question in her mind or reasonable doubt that the description is unclear, to review the document with both management's designated representative and the worker's representative in the event that questions may arise later after the position is filled. If this precaution is not taken, the possibility exists that the worker may file a complaint with the shop steward. Also, if a worker is requested to perform a task or engage in an activity other than is specified in her job description, she may report that request to the shop steward, who would follow the complaint procedure. This could result in time taken from patient care. In accordance with union policy, if the worker in question neglects or would prefer not to enter a complaint, one of her peers may be inclined to do so for her. This is considered by the union worker not only as a personal protective mechanism but also as an assurance that the terms of the union contract, which include the job description, are being upheld by both labor and management. In the past, managers have covered the unspecified, vague areas of the job description with the blanket phrase "whatever else deemed necessary." It would be much more appropriate and acceptable to include an emergency phrase and to define what constitutes an emergency.

In nursing, it is often difficult to determine when and with whom activities begin and end. This fine line will depend not only upon the wording of a job description, as mentioned earlier, but on the response or attitude of the workers involved. The worker's attitude has a direct effect on the patient and the care he receives, particularly if nurses draw fine lines between what they can do and what they will do for the patient. These lines are often obvious: vital signs are taken by aides, medications are administered by registered nurses, and treatments are performed by the technical nurse (LPN). But if this area of the contract is not carefully worded and clearly explained to the workers, the patient becomes the victim.

If unionization exists in your agency, it is the responsibility of the nurse-manager to handle the gray areas that arise in a way that is acceptable and agreeable to the majority involved and to the patient in particular. If she cannot resolve the problem, she must use the channels designated by the contract. The patient at no time should be aware that a union that exists in the agency is causing any disruption among staff members.

Conflicts can also arise as a result of personality differences. These conflicts must be handled on an individual basis. If a segment of the nursing staff is organized, such as the nursing assistants, and the professional staff is not, there is a possibility that the professionals unknowingly will make requests of the organized workers that are not included in the workers' agreement. If this is not resolved quickly and with a degree of diplomacy, a split will occur among staff members. It is essential for those persons working with organized staff members to understand the content and specific limitations of the contract in relation to work responsibilities. In some hospitals, the personnel director is the person management has designated to handle labor relations. He should be familiar with the contract content in order that he can readily interpret contractual terminology so that it can be understood by both union and nonunion employees. Concern for a smooth-working organization and the assurance that quality patient care is given should be uppermost in the minds of all parties.

Frequently, in the heat of negotiation and the bargaining process, these concerns are lost or misplaced, and personal gratification and personality dominance take precedence. It is here that both labor and management must be objective and open-minded. The test of a union contract should not be who is getting the most and who is giving the least but is this contract one in which a framework for a good, sound working relationship for all parties will evolve.

FACTORS THAT INVITE UNIONIZATION

In addition to the geographic location, size of hospital, preparation of staff, influx of patients and a myriad of other factors, five factors are probably the most basic reasons why unionization takes place.

Poor Patient Care

Poor patient care is self-explanatory. A professional nurse who is concerned will not tolerate poor or unsafe practices. If she has exhausted all her alternatives in an attempt to bring the problem to the attention of her supervisor, she may believe that she has no recourse short of resignation to resolve her problem except to consider unionization. This alternative solution is emphasized by union representatives when they sense an undercurrent of dissatisfaction among staff members and the possibility that a nonunion nursing service is considering unionization. Union representatives stress with the distraught employee that they can provide answers that will usually guarantee the employee that through their intervention, the patient's needs will be met. Possible solutions to avoid this stress factor are available to management: how often they review their philosophy (and is it actually being carried out?); the quality assurance programs (are they effective?); the lines of communication (are they open?). Time must be taken to evaluate.

Lack of Adequate Staff

"Never enough people to cover" is a familiar remark, but doing something about inadequate staffing is another matter, as was discussed in Chapter 9. One error that is frequently made in nursing administration is a lack of sharing the reasons for the staffing problems. Why the shortage? What is its cause? How long will it exist? Is there an end in sight? Nurses are by nature patient people, and very concrete thinkers. Give them some answers. If the nurse does not get them from her leaders, she'll seek them elsewhere, or allow the not knowing to increase frustration to the point where she will be a willing participant in union activities.

Salary Scale

With the continual increase in the cost of living it is common practice for employees anxiously to await that cost of living increase or merit increase or shift differential. If any or all of the expected increments are denied without an explanation that is within reason and satisfies the employee, again the accessibility of the union will not be overlooked.

Low Morale

The attitude that exists among staff can be likened to an epidemic: if it hits one, it can spread and infect an entire populace, in this case a nursing staff. As described in Chapter 8, motivation and attitude walk hand in hand. The absence of motivation leads to a negative attitude. This too will cause restlessness, dissatisfaction, and a "look to others" for the answers. Reasons for low morale are many and varied, but frequently a good starting point to search for the answers is the attitude of top-level managers in the agency.

Lack of Participation

No one likes to be left out. Today in most of our activities, we look to others for their opinions, suggestions, and approval or acceptance. A nursing staff is no different. If a professional nurse, as staff worker, is expected to perform certain activities/functions, she should have the opportunity to express her feelings and make recommendations. A representative from the group that is the informal leader (described in Chapter 4) can often prevent internal disruption that could lead to unionization. Listen to her.

Preventive measures are work tools that should be used daily in the health care setting by managers. If the preventive measures that have been described can be applied prior to any staff disruption, the prospects of unionization in a health care agency can be minimized, if not totally avoided.

LABOR RELATIONS AND THE NURSE-MANAGER

Today the nursing administrator must be programmed to be a knowledgeable participant in contract negotiation. In order to do this, there are specific areas related to unionization that she must become cognizant of. In 1977, Fralic (5) listed and described nine of these areas:

1. Know the basics of the NLRA.
2. Review the National Labor Relations Board (NLRB) certification.
3. Arrange for didactic preparation.
4. Utilize consultants and resources as needed.
5. Anticipate demands that will be made.
6. Plan for selective and systematic reading of latest literature.
7. Develop a new vocabulary.
8. Consider your emotional investment.
9. Plan for the possibility of a strike.

Each area should be given equal attention by the nurse-manager if she is successfully to involve herself in any negotiations.

1. *Know the NLRA.* Certainly the nurse-manager should not be expected to understand every facet of NLRA, but she must have a basic understanding of the role she will play in the event that unionization is expected to or does occur in her agency. She must know specifically what is contained in the contract that could affect her decision-making process and the functions of her department.

2. *Review the NLRB certification.* The nurse-manager must know who in her specific agency is the legally appointed representative in the contract negotiations and interpretation of contract content.

3. *Arrange for formal didactic preparation.* The nurse-manager should attend seminars and workshops that will familiarize her with the entire bargaining process. She cannot work with a union if she does not understand what it is and how it functions.

4. *Utilize consultants and resources.* There should be no hesitation on the manager's part to call upon experts to aid in expanding her knowledge of labor relations. If she is familiar with the process, she can often avoid pitfalls. She should profit by the experience of others who either have unions or have had experience with threat of unionization. The nurse-manager cannot be too well informed.

5. *Anticipate demands.* This area should be intuitive for the nurse-manager. She must know what to expect no matter how well the staff seems to be functioning. Be alert. Cues are always there, waiting to be recognized. Don't ignore them.

6. *Plan for selective reading of the latest literature.* Once you are knowledgeable about the topic of labor relations, do not put the books away. Read all the current literature available. The process is changing every day.

7. *Develop a new vocabulary.* The nurse-manager must be able to talk in union terms, to understand what is meant by grievance, negotiation, discrimination, and interference. Read not only the agency's contract, if one exists, but others that are available within and outside the health care industry.

8. *Consider your emotional investment.* The nurse-manager has a great deal at stake. In her position, she must set aside any personal feeling when she becomes involved in unionization. The staff she works with is the same one she has worked with in the past. She must be objective. To show antagonism would break down any chance for a workable relationship. The ultimate concern is the patient and his care.

9. *Plan for the possibility of a strike.* Be prepared, it could happen.

However, it is specifically stated in the NLRA that a 10-day notice is required. Take that time and use it wisely. Plan ahead. Meet with nursing supervisors, the administrator of the hospital, and other department heads that may be involved so that, if the strike should occur, a plan of action can be implemented immediately (5).

What has been discussed in this chapter merely scratches the surface. To consider all aspects of the topic of labor relations, unions, and unionization would and has filled many well-written books and periodicals. The main concern of all members of the health care field should be, not only how can we prevent unionization from occurring, which is of primary importance, but, in the event that unionization does occur, what can management do to maintain a cohesive relationship with the workers and foster a climate that will assure quality patient care.

REFERENCES

1. Pointer DD, Metzger N: *The National Labor Relations Act, A Guidebook for Health Care Facility Administrators.* New York, Spectrum Publications Inc., 1975, p. 1.
2. Sargis NM: Will nursing directors' attitude affect future collective bargaining? *J Nurs Adm* 8:25–26, December 1978.
3. Samaras JT: Administrative attitudes on collective bargaining in hospitals. *Supervisor Nurse* 9:59, January 1978.
4. Werther WB Jr, Lockhart CA: Collective action and cooperation in the health professions. *J Nurs Adm* 7:19, July-August 1977.
5. Fralic MF: The nurse director prepares for labor negotiations. *J Nurs Adm* 7:5–6, July-August 1977.

BIBLIOGRAPHY

Periodicals

Bryant YN: Labor relations in health care institutions: an analysis of Public Law 93-360. *J Nurs Adm* 8:28, March 1978.
Cleland US: Shared governance in a professional model of collective bargaining. *J Nurs Adm* 8:39, May 1978.
Donnelly G, et al: The anatomy of a conflict. *Supervisor Nurse,* p. 28, November 1975.
Emerson WL: Appropriate bargaining units for health care professional employees. *J Nurs Adm* 8:10, September 1978.

Erickson EH: Collective bargaining: an inappropriate technique for professionals. *J Nurs Adm* 3:54, March-April 1973.

Fralic MF: The nursing director prepares for labor relations. *J Nurs Adm* 7:4–8, July-August 1977.

Grand NK: Nursing ideologies and collective bargaining. *J Nurs Adm* 3:29, March-April 1973.

Helm EB: Negotiating a professional nurse's contract. *Hospital Topics* 56:24–28, March-April 1978.

Kravit S: Collective bargaining for professionals. *Supervisor Nurse* 4:46, July 1973.

Leininger M: The leadership crisis in nursing: a critical problem and challenge. *J Nurs Adm* 4:28, March-April 1974.

Metzger N: Labor relations: recent statistics show reversed trend toward unionization. *Hospitals* 52:115–120, April 1978.

Natonski J: Why a union contract didn't work at our hospital. *RN* 41:69–71, May 1978.

Reece DA: Union decertification and the salaried approach (a working alternative). *J Nurs Adm* 7:20, July-August 1977.

Rostowsky RD: Decentralization: innovation in management. *Hospital Topics* 56:14–16, September-October 1978.

Samaras JT: Administrative attitudes on collective bargaining in hospitals. *Supervisor Nurse* 9:56, January 1978.

Sargis NM: Will nursing directors' attitudes affect future collective bargaining? *J Nurs Adm* 8:21, December 1978.

Shepard IM: Health care institution labor law: case law developments, 1974–1978. *Am J Law in Medicine* 4:1–14, Spring 1978.

Werther WB Jr, Lockhart CA: Collective action and co-operation in the health professions. *J Nurs Adm* 7:13, July-August 1977.

Wynne D: A union contract was the only language our hospital would understand. *RN* 41:66–68, May 1978.

Books

Alexander EL: *Nursing Administration in the Hospital Health Care System,* ed 2. The CV Mosby Co, St Louis, 1978, pp. 51–57.

Pointer DD, Metzger N: *The National Labor Relations Act, A Guidebook for Health Care Facility Administrators.* New York, Spectrum Publications Inc, 1975.

Sloane AA, Witney F: *Labor Relations,* ed 2. Englewood Cliffs, NJ, Prentice-Hall Inc, 1972.

Stevens WF: *Management and Leadership in Nursing.* New York, McGraw-Hill Book Co, New York, 1978.

Appendix A: Job Description (Sample)

The content of the job description will vary, depending on the position that is being described. The philosophy of the agency and its size and type may also affect content. The suggested format below does encompass all areas that are relevant in describing a position totally.

Job Description*

Position Title	Department	Subdivision	Work Area
Supervisor—Days	Nursing	Nsg. Adm.	Med./Surg. Units

Job Summary. Provides and improves patient care by managing and evaluating the care rendered on the specified units; develops the managerial, clinical teaching and evaluation abilities of head nurses in these units; and is accountable for all nursing activities that are a direct or indirect responsibility.

Line of Authority	Areas of Directed Activities
Asst. Director—Nsg. Service	GN, 1N, 2N, 3N, 2W, 3W

*Permission has been granted by the Crozer-Chester Medical Center, Chester, Pennsylvania, to reproduce this format and the adapted content.

Specific Duties and Responsibilities.   In accordance with approved policies, procedures, and schedules of the hospital and nursing service:

I. Administer nursing services in specified areas.
  A. Activities to promote patient care
   1. Observes and evaluates adherence to established policies and standards of patient care through direct observation of care, records, reports, conferences, and committee meetings.
     a. Evaluates the response of patients to care.
     b. Evaluates nursing care plans.
     c. Assists the head nurse in developing and implementing effective plans for patient care and in solving nursing-care problems.
     d. Directs the head nurse in the use of resources to research and develop studies for the improvement of patient care.
     e. Observes and evaluates the performance of private duty nurses and makes recommendations as to their capabilities in specific assignments.
   2. Informs assistant director—nursing service of the progress of patients, patient care problems, and planned course of action.
   3. Encourages flexible and creative approaches to nursing care for patients and makes recommendations to head nurses and assistant director.
  B. Evaluates and determines with the head nurses the quality and quantity of nursing personnel needed to render nursing care based on patient needs, unit census, and budget controls.
   1. Interprets staffing policies, patterns, and mix to head nurses.
   2. Works with coordinators of staffing and other supervisors in the implementation and evaluation of the variable staffing technique.
   3. Confers daily with coordinators of staffing on staffing needs, analyzes and plans with the coordinators and other supervisors the resolution of any problems. Informs head nurses of changes in assignments.
   4. Obtains from the coordinators of staffing the names of per diem personnel assigned to weekend and weekday coverage for each four-week schedule. Informs head nurses of personnel assigned to their units.
  C. Assists the assistant director—nursing service in the planning, implementation, and evaluation of studies of staffing and staff-

ing patterns in specified areas. Formulates recommendations
to the director of nursing.

II. Supervisory responsibilities
   A. Directs head nurses in the management of units.
      1. Defines and interprets to head nurses their role and func-
         tions in relation to all personnel within the nursing depart-
         ment, hospital administration, medical staff, other depart-
         ments and personnel, and patients and families.
      2. Directs head nurses in the implementation and evaluation
         of approved unit policies and procedures for the delivery of
         nursing care, communications, staff scheduling, and main-
         tenance of records, reports, and manuals.
      3. Develops and maintains a free flow of written and oral
         communications between and among head nurses.
      4. Assists the head nurses in interpreting audits and results
         (outcomes) pertaining to their units and in developing a
         plan of action to resolve problems.
      5. Interprets to head nurses approved or changed personnel
         policies for employment, as described in the personnel
         handbook, as well as those for leave of absence, lateness,
         sick time.
      6. Interviews applicants for head nurse positions in specified
         areas and makes recommendations to assistant director.
      7. Guides head nurses in the use of approved tools for mea-
         suring the performance of nursing staff and in planning
         for periodic evaluation of personnel.
      8. Guides and directs head nurses in the administration and
         evaluation of the tools and in interpreting the outcomes to
         the nursing staff.
      9. Assists head nurses in establishing annual goals for the
         unit and programming approaches to their implementa-
         tion and evaluation. Encourages the attainment of goals
         and gives recognition for those attained.
     10. Develops standards and tools for and evaluates the per-
         formances of head nurses. Informs assistant director—
         nursing service of recommended action. Develops a sched-
         ule for periodic evaluation of performance of head nurses.
     11. Provides head nurses with the information needed to un-
         derstand their role in budget planning.
   B. Staff education
      1. Determines needs for staff development through direct ob-
         servation, consultation with head nurses, nursing staff,

medical staff, chairmen of standing committees of the nursing service organization, and evaluation of records and reports. Makes recommendations to assistant director.
2. Develops the head nurses' expertise in the application of management and teaching principles.
3. Provides programs for the continued managerial and teaching functions of head nurses (management principles and techniques, training and development of employees, decision making and problem solving, fiscal planning, effective employee relations, and clinical expertise).
4. Identifies the head nurses' responsibility for unit inservice programs and staff attendance at general inservice programs. Assists head nurses in implementing policies for attendance and use of tools for evaluation of the effectiveness of programs.
5. Conducts, with the assistance of the inservice department, the orientation program for all newly appointed head nurses on specified units. Provides for evaluation of the program and makes recommendations to assistant director.
6. Recommends the acquisition of books for unit libraries to the assistant director—nursing service and inservice education.
C. Environment
1. Maintains an environment conducive to the welfare of patients, staff, and visitors.
a. Involves head nurses in the development, implementation, and evaluation of policies and procedures for the safety and welfare of patients and staff.
b. Determines, with the head nurses, the quality or equipment and supplies needed to render safe patient care in specified units.
c. Conducts planned and impromptu periodic safety checks on each unit.
d. Works with supervisory personnel in other departments to resolve environmental problems.
e. Uses resource people and library resources to increase knowledge and understanding of safety codes.
2. Interprets patient and personnel environmental needs to assistant director—nursing service and recommends revisions, additions, and/or deletions.
III. Administrative responsibilities
A. Contributes to the development and evaluation of the philosophy and objectives of nursing service; interprets the philoso-

phy and objectives to head nurses; and utilizes the philosophy and objectives in planning, implementing, controlling, and evaluating all methods and/or systems for the delivery of nursing care.

B. Implements approved studies to identify nursing personnel and patient care problems, assists assistant director — nursing service in evaluating findings, and participates in formulation of recommendations to director of nursing.

C. Analyzes and approves all incidents, medication-intravenous errors, evaluation reports, and records prior to forwarding them to assistant director — nursing service.

   1. Adheres to system established in nursing service for the maintenance of all reports and records.

   2. Works with all supervisors to collect data on all incidents, medication-intravenous errors, and pressure-area reports; and submits to the assistant director — nursing service a summary of each type of report quarterly and an annual summary of each by specified date.

   3. Notifies director — nursing service of any incidents, errors, and evaluation reports that require the director's immediate knowledge and action.

D. Evaluates justification for overtime prior to approving the head nurses' request for staff to work overtime. Signs all overtime forms, indicating the reason(s), prior to submitting them to assistant director — nursing service.

E. Administration of budget for assigned units.

   1. Interprets to head nurses their responsibility for control of the budget.

   2. Assists assistant director — nursing service in the preparation of budget schedules.

   3. Analyzes monthly budget reports for each unit, obtains reasons for discrepancies from head nurses, delegates to head nurses the responsibility for making corrections, and reports findings and plan of action to assistant director — nursing service.

F. Makes the head nurses aware of their accountability for quality patient care.

G. Establishes goals for the improvement of patient care and nursing service, interprets goals to head nurses, and evaluates self-ability to fulfill goals.

H. Maintains intra-interdepartmental relationships for effective functioning of nursing service and all other departments.

   1. Confer at established time with representatives from the

following departments to discuss mutual problems, plans of action, and follow-up: x-ray, laboratory, medical records, physical medicine, pharmacy, escort service, heart station, respiratory therapy, and discharge planning.

   2. Obtains from and informs other supervisors of problems, involves them in plan of action, evaluation of findings, and recommendations for resolution of problems.

   3. Confers with assistant director—nursing service on recommendations prior to presenting them to departmental representatives.

I. Evaluates records and forms used to record nursing care and makes recommendations to appropriate personnel and/or committee chairman.

J. Contributes to patient care through membership and active participation on hospital, medical, and nursing service committees.

K. Consults with other supervisors—days in planning personal time schedules to avoid conflict in holiday and vacation plans and every-other-weekend coverage.

L. Keeps abreast of trends in nursing and nursing practice through attendance at workshops, conferences, seminars, and utilization of library resources.

M. Assists in interpreting nursing and nursing practice to nursing staff, medical staff, and other departmental personnel, and the community.

N. Reports to assistant director—nursing service and, in the absence of assistant director—nursing service, to a designated person.

Qualifications: (1) Graduate of an approved school of nursing. (2) Current licensure. (3) Baccalaureate degree in nursing with additional courses in management principles preferred; baccalaureate degree in business administration will be considered; at least four years of nursing experience, including two years as a head nurse, required.

Described by   **Approved by**   **Date of Approval**   **Date of**
                                                     Reevaluation
                                           of Job Description

---

Appendix B: Patient Questionnaire (Sample)

Quality Assurance and Accountability

The content of the patient questionnaire will vary from one facility to another depending on type of facility, length of patient's stay, and agency's philosophy. However, the content described should contain information necessary to determine overall quality care and accountability in most facilities.

	Yes	No	Not Appli- cable
1. Was your admission process smooth and well organized?	——	——	——
2. Were you escorted to your room immediately after admission process? If not, what was the waiting period? _____	——	——	——
3. Were you introduced to the staff and your roommates?	——	——	——
4. Was a history taken by the nurse?	——	——	——
5. How long did this procedure take? _____			
6. Were all hospital tests explained to you prior to having them done? If not, which ones were not explained? _____	——	——	——
7. Was the room equipment explained to you—for example, bed, call system, television, telephone, and so forth?	——	——	——

	Yes	No	Not Appli-cable
8. If surgery was involved, were you told what time the procedure would take place and what the presurgery preparations would be?	——	——	——
9. Was the food served in an appealing manner?	——	——	——
10. Was ample time given to eat your food?	——	——	——
If you were on a special diet, was it explained to you?	——	——	——
11. If you were unable to manage your food, were you offered assistance?	——	——	——
12. If pain medications were ordered, did you have to ask for them?	——	——	——
Were they offered to you?	——	——	——
13. If you had a need for assistance, was it offered to you?	——	——	——
Did you have to request assistance?	——	——	——
14. Did the staff appear to be aware of the information given to you by the physician — for example, "May I get out of bed? May I go to the bathroom?"	——	——	——
15. If you needed the services of other departments, such as x-ray, physical therapy, or respiratory therapy, was this explained to you by the nurse prior to the treatment?	——	——	——
16. If your physical problem required follow-up assistance at home, were the procedures explained to your family?	——	——	——
Were they demonstrated to your family, if necessary?	——	——	——
17. As time of discharge approached, were you given enough time to make the necessary preparation?	——	——	——

If so, how much time? _____

(days, hours)

	Yes	*No*	*Not Appli- cable*
18. Did your physician explain to you the limitations, if any, in your activities prior to or at the time of discharge?	——	——	——
19. If medications, prescriptions, or supplies were needed for your care at home, were they available to you at time of discharge?	——	——	——

INDEX

Achievement motivation, 94
Accountability, 31, 35, 120
  decentralization and, 29-30
  responsibility distinguished from, 24
Actualization needs, 91
Administrative structure, *see*
    Organizational structure of health
    care agencies
Advocacy, 34-35
Aggression, 96
American Nurses Association's
    Standards for Nursing Practice, 132
Audit, quality care and, 33-34
Authority, leadership with, 40
  leadership without, 39-40
  organizational structure and levels of,
    14
Autocratic leadership style, 42-46

Behavior modification, 94
Belonging needs, 90
Board of trustees, budgeting process and,
    148, 149
Budgets (budgeting), 144-167
  capital, 149-150, 164-167
  monthly, 161-163
  objectives of, 149
  operating, 149-150
  period for, 150
  preparation of, 151-160
  types of, 149-150
Bureaucratic leadership style, 44
Bureaucratic model, 16

Capital budget, 149-150, 164-167
Care sharing, 30
Case nursing, 108

CAT scanners, 146
Centralization, 29
  see also Decentralization
Change, 75-84
  concept of, 76
  job description and, 126
  methods of, 76-77
  resistance to, 78-80
Change objectives, 8
Change process: first phase of, 77-78
  second phase of, 78-84
  third phase of, 84
Communication, 50-61
  eliminating barriers to effective, 57-61
  inter-intra departmental, 60-61
  job description and, 128
  motivation and, 99
  organizational structure and, 14
  words and language and, 51-57
Compensation, 97
Confrontation-negotiation leadership
    style, 43
Consumerism, quality care and, 27
Contractual relationships, 20
Controller, 148-149
Cooperative relationship, 20
Coordinating relationship, 20
Costs of health care, 145-147
  behavior of, 150
  quality care and, 25-27
  staffing and, 105-106

Decentralization, 29-30
Defensive behaviors, 96-97
Democratic leadership style, 43, 45, 46
Directive approach, 56-57
Displacement, 97

Division of labor, 14

Emotions, persuasion through, 81
  problem-solving process and, 72
Employment variables, job description
  and, 124
Esteem needs, 90-91
Evaluation, *see* Staff evaluation
Expectancy model of motivation, 94

Fair Labor Standards Act, 145
Federal government, staffing and,
  106-107
Fiscal planning, *see* Budgets (budgeting)
Fixed costs, 150
Flat organization structure, 29
Fringe benefits, 109-110
Frustration, 96
Functional method of patient
  assignment, 108

Goals of health care agencies, 2-3

Health care agencies, 1-22
  objectives of, 6-8
  organizational structure of, *see*
    Organizational structure of health
    care agencies
  philosophy of, 3-5, 107
  policies and procedures of, 8-11
  purpose and goals of, 2-3
  recent changes in, 145-146
Hierarchy, 16-18
  see also Organizational structure of
    health care agencies

Improvement objectives, 8
Individuality, communication and, 57
Inflation, 26-27
Influence, change process and, 81
Informal leadership, 39-40
Informal organizational structure, 20-22
Information, problem-solving process
  and, 71, 72
Informative presentation, 56-57
Insurance, health care, 26
Interruptions, communication and, 58
Interview, staff evaluation and, 139-140

Job descriptions, 118-129, 133
  administrative advantages of, 127-129

definition of, 119
formats for, 121-124
inside consultation or outside
  consultation in writing, 120
unionization and, 172-173
utilization of, 125-127
Job knowledge, 124
Job summary, 121-123
Job title, 121
Joint Commission on Accreditation for
  Hospitals (JCAH), 24

Labor-management relations, 168-178
  nurse-managers and, 176-178
  see also Unionization
Laissez-faire leadership style, 43, 45-46
Leadership, 37-47
  effective, 41-42
  formal and informal, 39-40
  management and, 38-39
  problem-solving approaches and, 42
  staffing, and 112-115
  styles of, 37-38, 42-47
Legislation, 106
Line relationships, 14-15
Listening, 52-53
Long-range objectives, 7
Love needs, 90

Maintenance objectives, 8
Management, leadership and, 38-39
  McGregor's Theory X and Theory Y of,
    92-93
  participative theory of, 93
  scientific, 88
  unions and, 169-170
  see also Labor-management relations
Management by objectives (MBO)
  approach, 7
Managers, primary relationships
  among, 60
Manipulation, 39
Matrix structure, 16-18
Medicare, 145
Monistic theory of motivation, 88
Monthly budget, 161-163
Morale, productivity and, 93
  unionization and, 175-176
Motivation, 87-101, 111
  achievement, 94
  application of theories of, 94-95

behavioral considerations and, 95-97
definition of, 95
expectancy model of, 94
Herzberg's theory of, 91-92
hierarchy of needs theory of, 88-89
Likert's theory of, 93
McGregor's Theory X and Theory Y
     of, 92-93
monistic theory of, 88
nurse-managers and, 97-101

National Labor Relations Act (NLRA),
     168-169, 177, 178
National Labor Relations Board
     (NLRB), 168-169, 177, 178
Needs, hierarchy of, 88-91
Noise, communication and, 58
Nursing rounds, 31-32

Objectives of health care agencies, 6-8
Occupational Safety and Health Act
     OSHA), 28
Open-door policy, 60-61
Operating budget, 149-150
Organizational chart, 18-20
Organizational philosophy, of health
     care agencies, 3-5
Organizational structure of health
     care agencies, 13-22
  diagram of, 18-20
  flat, 29
  informal, 20-22
  line and staff relationships, 14-15
  pyramid and matrix structures, 15-18
  quality care and, 27-30
  reasons for, 14
Orientation, job description and, 125
Outcome objectives, 7
Oversimplification, problem-solving
     and, 70-71
Overthinking, 59

Participative management theory, 93
Patient advocate, quality care and, 34-35
Patient assignments, staffing and,
     107-109
Payroll, budget preparation and, 158-164
Peer review, 136
  quality care and, 32-33
Performance descriptions, 133
Permanent objectives, 7

Personality, problem-solving process
     and, 71
Persuasion, change and, 80-81
Philosophy of health care agencies, 3-5
  staffing patterns and, 107
Physician's assistant (PA), 19
Placating, problem-solving process and,
     73
Policies of health care agencies, 8-11
Positive reinforcement, 94, 97
Preparation, level of, 124
Primary nursing, 105-106, 108-109
Primary relationships among managers,
     60
Problem-solving, 63-73
  awareness of problems and, 64
  labor-management relations and, 172
  leaders' approach to, 42
  obstacles to, 69-73
  steps in process of, 64-69
Procedures, 11
Process objectives, 7
Productivity, morale and, 93
Professional Standards Review
     Organizations (PSROs), 24, 106, 132
Promotions, job descriptions and, 126
Purposes of health care agencies, 2-3
Pyramid structure, 16, 18

Qualifications, job descriptions and,
     123-124
Quality assurance, 23-25
  definition of, 23-24
  nursing staff and, 31-35
  stff evaluation and, 132-133
Quality care, care sharing and, 30
  Consumerism and, 27
  cost and, 25-27
  job description and, 127
  nursing staff and, 31-35
  organization complexity and, 27-30
  staffing and, 104
Questionnaires, quality assurance and,
     33

Rationalization, 97
Reason, persuasion through, 80-81
Regression, 97
Repression, 97
Responsibility, 24
Role expansion, quality care and, 35

Rounds, nursing, 31-32

Safety needs, 90
Salary, qualifications and, 123-124
Salary scale, unionization and, 175
Schedules, staffing and, 109, 114-115
Scientific management, 88
Self-esteem, motivation and, 88, 90
Self-fulfillment, 89, 91
Semivariable costs, 150
Short-range objectives, 7
Staff evaluation, 127, 131-141
 disagreement of employee with, 141
 distortions in, 138
 interview and, 139-140
 methods for, 137-138
 by nurse-managers, 136
 by peers, 136
 purposes of, 133-134
 quality assurance and, 132-133
 scheduling of, 134-136
 trait language *versus* event language, 137
Staffing (staffing patterns), 104-115
 availability of care providers and, 110-111
 budget preparation and, 152, 155
 conventional, 113-114
 cost of health care and, 105-106
 cyclic, 113-114
 fringe benefits and, 109-110
 job description and, 128-129
 leadership and, 112-115
 length of stay of employees and, 111-112

patient assignments and, 107-109
 scheduling and, 109, 114-115
 7-day on, 7-day off, 114
 team, 115
 12-hour plan, 114-115
 type and location of facility and, 110
Staff relationships, 14-15
Standards for Nursing Practice American Nurses Association), 132
Stress, problem-solving and, 69-70
Structure objectives, 6-7
Survival needs, 89

Team nursing, 108
Team staffing, 115
Theory X, 92
Theory Y, 92-93

Unionization, 168-170
 factors that invite, 174-176
 patient care and, 172-174
Unions, attitudes of management toward, 169-170

Variable costs, 150

Withdrawal, 96-97
Wordiness, 59
Words, communication and, 51-57
Working environment, job description and, 124
Work schedules, staffing and, 109, 114-115